YOUR DOCTOR IS WRONG

methods that just cover over the symptoms (or produce serious side effects!) actually get results based on our natural body's physiology and chemistry. A must-read if you want to survive the current conventional medical system, and have vibrant health!"

—**Hyla Cass MD, author of** *8 Weeks to Vibrant Health*.

"Don't treat the symptoms, treat the source!" is the message I took away from Dr. Norling's book. Medical care has become so fractured into its various specialty areas, that patients can sometimes get lost in the shuffle. Dr. Norling shows us how to put the pieces of the puzzle back together through her Functional Medicine approach. Treating the whole person is foundational to her model."

—**R.W. "Chip" Watkins, MD, MPH, FAAFP,
Chief Medical Officer Sanesco International.**

"Sharon Norling is a shining star in the new medicine. She brings laughter, joy and healing to all who see her. Read this book and benefit from her experience."
—**Gregory A. Plotnikoff, MD, MTS, FACP Co-author:** *Trust Your Gut.*

"Dr. Norling's book may be seen as controversial because some people will not like what she has to say…they will find it hard to believe until they see all the facts as Dr.Norling presents them. Her thought-provoking facts challenge our traditional thinking about 'right and wrong' choices in maintaining a healthy lifestyle. Exceptional!"

—**Kathleen FitzSimons, PhD**

"Dr. Norling systemically outlines the process to health, wholeness and transformation. Thinking outside the accepted 'norm' box is the only way to improve and take control of our own health. Your Doctor is Wrong is empowering! It's your path to optimal health."

—**David Villarreal, DDS Certified Biological Dentist (IABDM)**

"Very useful information! Presented simply and to the point; obviously the result of many years of careful investigation and clinical experience. Identify and treat the cause as opposed to merely suppressing symptoms. Giving the body what it needs and it will function as nature intended. Brilliant!"

—**Dr. Stephen M. Danielsen, N.D.**

"One of the primary responsibilities of any business owner is to constantly move their business forward—with new ideas, a bigger vision and unfailing energy for what they do. Unfortunately, for too many entrepreneurs, that kind of energy and mental focus isn't available once their health and emotional well-being is compromised. If you've been wondering what more you can do to achieve vibrant good health, superb mental acuity and abundant energy, then read Dr. Sharon Norling's book. It's a whole new approach to improving your health…and your bottom line."

—**Janet Switzer, International small-business authority and New York Times bestselling coauthor of**
The Success Principles: How to Get From Where You Are to Where You Want to Be.

"I was an addict for twenty years and thought it was more than a moral decision. Dr. Norling has helped me understand the bio-chemistry of the disease that plagued me for so long. This informative book has freed me even more. I praise her and her research. Fantastic information for anyone suffering from addiction or knows someone who is. Everyone should read this book…everyone."

—**John Roth**

"I am thrilled to recommend this book authored by my friend of over 30 years, Dr. Sharon Norling. You will find it as informative, inspirational and motivating, as she is in person. Dr. Norling's book will enrich and improve the quality of your life, now and for the rest of your life. I respect her incredible expertise in this field of advanced medicine. You will learn and benefit from reading Your Doctor is Wrong."

—**Sheila Cluff, Internationally renowned health and fitness expert.**

YOUR DOCTOR IS WRONG

*Survival Guide
for Dismissed,
Misdiagnosed or Mistreated*

Sharon Norling, MD, MBA

NEW YORK

YOUR DOCTOR IS WRONG
Survival Guide for Dismissed, Misdiagnosed or Mistreated

Published in New York, New York, by Morgan James Publishing. Morgan James and The Entrepreneurial Publisher are trademarks of Morgan James, LLC. www.MorganJamesPublishing.com

The Morgan James Speakers Group can bring authors to your live event. For more information or to book an event visit The Morgan James Speakers Group at www.TheMorganJamesSpeakersGroup.com.

This book contains advice and materials relating to one's health care. It is not to replace any medical advice by your physician and should only be used to supplement rather than replace care by your doctor. All efforts have been made to assure accuracy of the information contained in this book as of the date of publication. The publisher and the author disclaim any liability for any medical outcomes that may occur as a result of applying the methods suggested in this book. It is highly recommended that you seek your physician's advice before starting on any medical program or treatment.

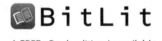

A FREE eBook edition is available
with the purchase of this print book

CLEARLY PRINT YOUR NAME IN THE BOX ABOVE

Instructions to claim your free eBook edition:
1. Download the BitLit app for Android or iOS
2. Write your name in UPPER CASE in the box
3. Use the BitLit app to submit a photo
4. Download your eBook to any device

ISBN 978-1-63047-077-7 paperback
ISBN 978-1-63047-078-4 eBook
ISBN 978-1-63047-079-1 hardcover
Library of Congress Control Number:
2013957726

Cover Design by:
Chris Treccani
www.3dogdesign.net

Interior Design by:
Bonnie Bushman
bonnie@caboodlegraphics.com

In an effort to support local communities, raise awareness and funds, Morgan James Publishing donates a percentage of all book sales for the life of each book to Habitat for Humanity Peninsula and Greater Williamsburg.

Get involved today, visit
www.MorganJamesBuilds.com

Habitat
for Humanity®
Peninsula and
Greater Williamsburg
Building Partner

DEDICATION

I would like to dedicate my book to two women in my life, who have had the wisdom of right and wrong, and know the strength we have in our choices.

Ella Ritz Norling, my mother…who taught me to never see barriers.

Bonnie Nyberg Hankinson, my friend…best friend since kindergarten, who has been there for me, through all my trials and tribulations, along with all my joys and celebrations.

CONTENTS

ACKNOWLEDGMENTS

First and foremost, I want to acknowledge my many patients who told me I had to write this book. You have taught me so much. It is your voice that needed to be heard. You inspire me and touch my heart. Thank you.

The credit for getting this book completed goes to Kate Marsh. Kate is a true professional. There isn't a job or a task she can't accomplish and accomplish it to perfection. As my assistant she always goes the extra mile. Her critical thinking, creativity and positive attitude are priceless. I am so very grateful for all that you do. Thank you so much.

Karen Czarske, our receptionist, is the foundation of my practice at the Mind Body Spirit Center. She held it all together as I dedicated the time and energy to write this book. Her sense of humor makes everyday fun. Karen's attention to detail is incredible. Her wisdom impresses me. My practice would not be what it is today without her. I am so grateful.

Ann K. Castle, my editor. Many thanks. You did a brilliant job of editing what I put in the book that didn't need to be there and what I omitted that did need to be written. I cherish your advice, friendship, and hard work. Your dedication to this book was outstanding.

A special thanks to Jack Canfield and Janet Switzer who taught me the Success Principles and motivated me to write this book. I want to acknowledge

Steve Harrison and the Quantum Leap staff for teaching me how to write a book. You taught me the importance of marketing so more people informed on how to stop their pain and suffering. Any shortcomings in this book are all mine and not a reflection of your work!

To Wendy Lipton-Dibner, you are an inspiration to me. Your Move People to Action and the Elite Video Mastery courses gave me the invaluable information and tools that I needed. Thank you and your speakers.

Toki Lee, an amazing photographer, thank you for capturing my essence in the photo. You are a joy to work with.

Thank you, thank you, Bonnie. Bonnie Hankinson, who supported me throughout this project—your encouragement and brilliant creativity is extraordinary. I know you are grateful that I didn't put any of our life stories in this book. That book will be my next bestseller!

I want acknowledge Sheila Cluff and Pam Price, both authors, and longtime friends who gave me the opportunity to see the world and medicine from a new perspective.

I am forever grateful to all my friends and family that encouraged my outrageous sense of humor some of which is reflected in this book. You know who you are. I want to give a very big thank you to my family who love and accept me for being an "out of the box" relative. A special thanks to my brother, Lefty, you are such a fantastic brother. I have learned so much from you.

My perspective on medicine and health has evolved over the years and I want to acknowledge the many physicians that contributed to my education and training. I want to express my respect for all the right physicians who have dedicated their lives giving their best care to patients.

Additionally, I want to credit my colleagues who have tried to discredit my ideas, my work, and occasionally, me personally. I understand that they have not been educated or trained in this field. Many, because of time constraints, have not been able to keep up on the literature. Some are not as open to change or new concepts. Whatever the reasons, they have made me wiser. They continue to inspire me to conduct research, attend many medical conferences each year, educate my patients, and give my best care to our mutual patients.

I want to acknowledge all the doctors who are bright, well-educated, up-to-date, dedicated and compassionate. You are the right doctors.

INTRODUCTION

My practice is filled with patients who have been dismissed, misdiagnosed and their symptoms have just been treated like the tip of the iceberg with a pharmaceutical drug.

This book has answers. It has facts. It has hope. Your Doctor is Wrong is written for the people who have been told "There's nothing wrong with you." What is really wrong is the doctor has not found the root cause of the illness.

It has hope for the patient who has been told "You will need to stay on this (pharmaceutical drug) for the rest of your life." Well, of course, you do when the doctor hasn't found the underlying cause or causes of the problem.

The case studies in this book are real-people. People I have personally cared for. They bring stories of suffering, transformation and optimism.

The number of deaths from medical errors will shock you. Remember these are the reported errors. I have been in medicine for over 30 years as a nurse, physician, medical school faculty, and vice president and senior management in large healthcare organizations. I have been a patient. I have been an advocate. Let me assure you those numbers are far from the truth. Many times the death certificate will read "natural causes".

"Medication errors are among the most common medical errors, harming at least 1.5 million people every year," as reported by the Institute of Medicine of the National Academies. The extra medical costs of treating drug-related injuries occurring in hospitals alone conservatively amount to $3.5 billion a year, and this estimate does not take into account lost wages and productivity or additional health care costs.

"The frequency of medication errors and preventable adverse drug events is cause for serious concern," said committee co-chair Linda R. Cronenwett, dean and professor, School of Nursing, University of North Carolina, Chapel Hill.

"Studies indicate that 400,000 preventable drug-related injuries occur each year in hospitals. Another 800,000 occur in long-term care settings, and roughly 530,000 occur just among Medicare recipients in outpatient clinics. The committee noted that these are likely underestimates."

This is according to the Institute of Medicine Board on Health Care Services Committee on Identifying and Preventing Medication Errors, Written by J. Lyle Bootman, Ph.D., Sc.D., (co-chair) Dean and Professor, University of Arizona College of Pharmacy, et al. (2006).

What this book is NOT: It is not about bashing doctors or the medical profession. There are many physicians who are right, who are compassionate and who are up to date with the literature.

As physicians we pride ourselves as scientists. We should be open to critical thinking and not be judgmental about new ways of thinking, new medicine, or new opportunities for patient care just because we never learned it in medical school or residency. Almost all physicians' Continuing Medical Education (required CME) is given at medical conferences that are sponsored by pharmaceutical drug companies or biotech firms. We need to be open to learning other evidence-based medicine.

So how did I get "here"?

My medical career began as a nurse at St. Mary's School of Nursing (Mayo Clinic) in Rochester, Minnesota. Later I decided to become a physician. This wasn't an ordinary path.

I was married with three children, starting out as a freshman in college at age 28. After taking two classes in night school at Cleveland State University I made an appointment to see Dr. Caughey at Case Western Reserve University School of Medicine. He was chairman of the admissions committee.

I told him my story. He said, "Skip the first two years of college and start as a junior." I thought, "Well, that's a unique approach." I went back to Cleveland State University and registered my second quarter as a junior. Well, I tried. They explained that a college student needed to do their freshman year first, then sophomore and then junior.

Well, of course, I knew that. But I had my own plan. I asked to speak to the supervisor. The supervisor was a very serious lady and clearly had no sense of humor. She told me that under no uncertain terms could I start as a junior. I asked who the head of the Biology Department was and I was told it was Dr. John Morrison.

I went to see Dr. Morrison and, no surprises here he gave me the same answer. But I was stuck to that chair by Velcro. I was not moving. I told him my story why I needed to start as a junior, then he told me his story why that was not possible, then I told him my story, then he told me his story. We volleyed for a while… quite a while.

I finally said, "If I can't get the good grades that I need to get into medical school I will drop the junior classes and start over as a freshman." I think it was getting dark outside or he was getting hungry. He finally said, "Yes, you can start as a junior."

So now I was a junior. I had not had any math or chemistry for 14 years since I was in 9th grade high school algebra. I had never taken calculus, physics, or trigonometry. I was taking Bio-Chemistry without ever having taken college Biology or college Chemistry. I loved it! I was so excited to be on my path to become a doctor. I was filled with passion. The thought of me not being accepted into medical school never crossed my mind.

After finishing my junior year with a 3.8 GPA I went back to see Dr. Caughey. I told him I had followed his advice. He gave me early admission to medical school the following year. I needed to finish one more year of college. There were over 8,000 applications that year and he accepted 160 students. Years later I thought, "Why did he accept me?" Then I realized he had given me an "impossible" task and I completed it well. He also saw my determination, my tenacity, and my passion.

Graduating from medical school I wanted to be an OB/GYN. I was told, "You can't." I asked, "Why?" A Case Western University School of Medicine faculty then said, "Honey, you don't understand." As the surgeon patted me on the arm, he said, once again, "Honey, OB/GYN is a surgical subspecialty. You need to be able to stand on your feet and make a decision." He said, "A woman does not qualify." There were no women faculty members in the Department of OB/GYN. This was 1978.

I loved OB/GYN. I loved the acute care, deliveries, surgery, and the ER. Personally, I had been in the stirrups, I had 3 children, breast fed them and had GYN surgery. It was perfect for me. So I became an OB/GYN.

There are many, many stories of my life that brought me where I am today but I will save them for my next book.

After practicing OB/GYN for 12 years I was recruited to teach at the University of Minnesota Medical School. It was here that my life changed forever.

My family is from Minnesota. My wonderful sister-in-law, Pat, had breast cancer. She was dismissed and she was misdiagnosed. She had a breast mass and her doctor told her, "It is nothing. You are too young." I told her she needed to go to a surgeon and get it biopsied. The cancer had spread to her nodes. Reviewing the mammogram from the year before, a mass was present, but it had been missed.

I was her advocate. She was very interested in nutrition, massage, supplements, and spirituality. Clearly, no "well-educated" doctors knew anything about that. I went with her to her appointments and she asked, "What else can I do in addition to my surgeries, chemotherapy and radiation?" The physicians not only did not have the answer, but they didn't even respect the question.

After Pat died I vowed to do everything I could to change that. First, I had to learn "it". I made a commitment to learn this new medicine. My years at the university were transforming. I was on a sharp learning curve, as I had to stay one step ahead of the medical students and residents I was teaching this new medicine to.

My responsibilities included teaching, practicing gynecology, Medical Director of the OB/GYN Department's Women's Health Center, faculty at the Center for Spirituality and Healing, and a senior management position at the University Hospital and Clinics responsible for the 42 Ambulatory Care

Clinics. I lead the development of the Mind Body Spirit Clinic where we began to practice integrative and functional medicine.

Since I was in various leadership positions I thought it would be helpful to get a MBA. So I did. I had the opportunity to testify before the White House Commission on Complementary Alternative Medicine Policy and be a contributing author of a textbook, *Integrative Medicine*. During this time I was able to travel the world and I saw health care from an entirely new perspective. I began to realize that we had a lot to learn from other countries and cultures.

It was in the mid 90's when I first heard Jeffrey Bland, PhD, co-founder of the Institute of Functional Medicine speak at a seminar. I didn't understand a word he said. I only understood pharmaceutical conferences.

It was Jeffrey Bland and Functional Medicine that changed my life and I will be forever grateful. Functional Medicine is a comprehensive systems approach that cares for the whole person not just a body part. It uses specialty labs to find the underlying cause of illnesses and treats with lifestyle changes and evidenced-based natural products whenever possible. Once you start practicing functional medicine you can't go back.

My passion was steadfast. I had seen for many years' family, friends, and patients still suffering with chronic illnesses. They had no answers just new prescriptions.

Today I am board certified in OB/GYN, Integrative Medicine (ABIHM), and Medical Acupuncture (DABMA). I also have certifications in nutrition, biofeedback and Reiki.

I wrote this book because patients are still suffering. There are right tests, right answers, and right solutions. The chapters include patient stories, mainstream medical references, and are laced with humor.

You will find chronic illnesses caused by inflammation created from hidden IgG food allergies. The cause of heartburn and GERD can be diagnosed and treated instead of treating the tip of the iceberg with an antacid. The antacids can cause other chronic illnesses.

Questions about hormone health and safety are addressed. It's important to evaluate all the hormones and treat as indicated otherwise it is like sitting on a one legged stool. If you want to learn things you never knew about sex you might want to skip right over to Chapter 5. A new approach to addictions in Chapter 8 includes bio-chemical testing and targeted nutrient therapies.

Heart disease and its relationship to toxins are explored. Toxins and the dangers of personal skin care products, foods, and environments will grab your attention. You can't fix a problem unless you know what is causing it.

The last chapter asks the question, "Is the life you are living worth the life you are giving up?" This chapter encourages and empowers you. You will learn how to find the right doctor and be your own advocate.

This book can change your life forever. Nothing is more important than your health. Nothing.

This is not an ordinary book.

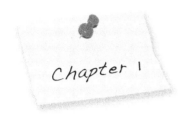

Chapter 1

MEDICALLY RIGHT
OR WRONG?

Each year 250,000 people die due to medical errors. That is equivalent to one and a half 747 jumbo jets crashing every day.

My mother had severe stomach pains. I remember her suffering as she lay on a small sofa in the living room at night trying not to disturb her family as she cried out in pain and we tried to sleep. She went to many doctors in our small rural Minnesota town as well as seeking help in Minneapolis and the Mayo Clinic. They told her, "There is nothing wrong with you." She was dismissed. She was misdiagnosed. They prescribed an antipsychotic medication, Thorazine. Within a year my mother died of stomach and esophageal cancer. She was 38 years old. I was 12.

Years later, my elderly father was diagnosed with colon cancer after months of a delayed diagnosis. He was healthy for his age and still had his great sense of humor. After surgery he never regained consciousness. I asked, "Why? What happened?" Even as a physician I never got an answer. "It could have been a stroke," I was told.

I stayed with him in the ICU for days. Then I went home to get some rest. After I fell asleep the phone rang. It was his doctor. Dr. M. told me my dad had died. Of course, I felt terrible. I wasn't there. I had left. I called my sons to ask them to be pallbearers. I dozed a little. In the early morning I called the hospital to let them know the name of the funeral home. I said, "I am calling about Stan Norling." The nurse said, "He is doing better, his blood pressure is up and he is stable."

The shock was unbelievable. To my horror I thought, did I dream this? I called my brother and said I had just talked to the hospital and dad was doing better. The look on his face can only be well described by my sister-in-law, Ruth Ann, who was standing next to him. The doctor had called him in the middle of the night and told him dad had died.

I drove 100 miles back to my hometown to see for myself. Dad was still alive in the ICU. His doctor left town that morning on vacation. He never ever called me or my brother back.

I suppose it goes without saying that a doctor should be able to determine if someone is dead or alive especially in the ICU.

Everyone has a story about someone they know or themselves who has been dismissed, misdiagnosed or their symptoms were just treated like the tip of the iceberg with a pharmaceutical drug.

Recent research published in the October issue 2012 of the *Annals of Family Medicine* show that chronic illness affects 45 percent of the US population and that 40 percent of people older than 60 years of age are now taking five or more medications. More medications are prescribed to alleviate the side effects of the already-prescribed medications.[1]

Pharmaceutical drugs inhibit, block or antagonize specific bio-chemical pathways. These are the very pathways that make your body work. What else do we know about pharmaceutical drugs?

- Medication errors are estimated to account for at least 7,000 deaths in the United States alone every year.[2]
- Over 770,000 patients are estimated to be injured because of medication errors every year.[3]

- The Food and Drugs Administration (FDA) in the United States says that at least 1 death occurs per day and 1.3 million people are injured each year due to medication errors.[4]
- Several studies point to more than 50 percent of potential and serious adverse events being associated with injectable medications.[5]
- One 5-year study showed that the most common types of medication errors were a wrong dose, a wrong drug or a wrong route of administration.[6]
- Medication errors occur in nearly 1 out of every 5 doses given to patients in the typical hospital.[7]
- Adverse medication events have been reported and are estimated to occur at a rate of around 5 percent for admissions and discharges from the typical hospital.[8]

According to the *New England Journal of Medicine*, medical care in the United States is uniformly mediocre. This report was one of the largest studies on health care quality in the U.S. It found that patients were found to receive proper care only 55 percent of the time. This study brought to light that no one is safe from poor quality medical care—myself included.

According to the August 14, 2013 issue of JAMA, US rankings relative to other countries got worse for:

- Death rate (from 18th to 27th)
- Years lost life (from 23rd to 28th)
- Years lived with disability (from 5th to 6th)
- Life expectancy at birth (from 20th to 27th)
- Healthy life expectancy (from 14th to 26th)

"The United States spends the most per capita on health care across all countries, lacks universal health coverage, and lags behind other high-income countries for life expectancy and many other health outcome measures."

Americans needlessly suffer and die at the hands of the medical establishment. No one, however, had ever analyzed all the published literature dealing with injuries and deaths caused by medicine.

That changed when a group of researchers meticulously reviewed the published statistical evidence and compiled a startling fully referenced report. According to the data compiled by these researchers, the number of people having adverse reactions to prescribed drugs in the hospital is 2.2. million per year.[9] The number of unnecessary antibiotics prescribed annually for viral infections is 20 million per year.[10,11] The number of unnecessary medical and surgical procedures performed annually is 7.5 million per year.[12] The number of people exposed to unnecessary hospitalization annually is 8.9 million per year.[13]

The most stunning statistic is the total number of deaths. An astounding 783,936 Americans die each year as a result of the medical care they receive. Today's medical system is the *leading cause of death and injury* in the U.S. By contrast, 577,190 deaths due to cancer and about 600,000 due to heart disease have been estimated for 2012.

Halstead Holman wrote in the *Journal of American Medical Association* that medicine is in need of new clinical education to better manage the rising prevalence of chronic disease.

Evaluating the whole person gives us whole answers. This method is a proven treatment that has worked for so many.

Most people wouldn't buy a car without checking consumer ratings, but they still rely largely on word of mouth to select a physician. Yet with more patients having to choose from a health plan's list, there is a growing demand for information that is more reliable than a friend's recommendation. It goes beyond the rudimentary details available online—a doctor's hours, educational background and ZIP code. Remember 50 percent of all doctors graduated in the bottom half of their class.

Aging baby boomers think 60 is the new 40. But 40 is not necessarily the benchmark of mature vigor or sound health. By age 35–40 men and women will probably already be suffering from a number of silent diseases.

Given the absence of significant conventional findings, these silent diseases and mild symptoms are overlooked or dismissed. Rather than finding the root cause early and preventing the progression, mainstream medicine treats full-blown diseases that may have been festering for years. Health insurance is like car insurance—you are only entitled to make a claim *after* a wreck, and then it may be too late.

Once you or your loved one has a serious disease or significant unbearable symptoms, all other issues become largely irrelevant. Your concern is how quickly I can get a relief in the least toxic way.

There is a better way. This book will give the direction, the help and the hope of living a longer, healthier life.

Every day in my practice I see patients who have been suffering with chronic illness for days, months, and even years. The conventional care practice is to recommend a prescription or do a surgery. How many times have you gone to your doctor and been told what to do and not been given options? Perhaps you were told, "It is all in your head," but you know you have symptoms. You know you are not well.

Are you are tired, anxious, depressed, can't focus, lack motivation, experience joint pain, can't sleep, have digestive issues and just don't feel well? If so, there is something wrong. The right doctor can find the root cause. To be a happy and successful person, health is a must.

You may have seen many doctors and spent the time, energy, and money looking for answers. Yet, all the routine tests come back negative. You look good on paper and have been told that there is nothing wrong with you because the doctor could not find the underlying cause.

Is the life you are living worth the life you are giving up?

Today we have a wide range of tests, from basic labs to sophisticated imaging that can be done to look for the root cause of symptoms or illnesses. The power of these tests in obtaining information and saving lives has encouraged the hope of a "magic bullet" for treatment; however this model has, to a large extent, failed to produce the same success with diseases that are multi-factorial and chronic in nature.

Illness starts because of a cause, illness continues because the cause continues, and illness can only be resolved when the cause is resolved.

You must find the underlying or root cause of an illness or a symptom rather than just treating the tip of the iceberg with a pharmaceutical drug. It is more than just taking a pill or having a procedure. Medicine is more than just naming a disease. It is more than a pill for an ill. You need and deserve to live your best life.

As education is often the key to health, keeping abreast of advances in medicine is critical, if challenging—even for physicians. In the past, physicians were taught to "blame or name" a disease. Unfortunately, according to the research, most doctors practice only what they have learned in medical school and residency. There's a huge gap between research and the way doctors practice. This is evident even in mainstream medical journals like the *Journal of American Medical Association*. "There is a large gap between what physicians do for patients with chronic diseases and what should be done."[14]

Today, we've learned that there is no such thing as a single disease, but rather the root causes of an illness that create diseases. If the underlying cause of a symptom is not identified and treated, disease or illness often occurs. This explains why people are often diagnosed with multiple diseases or symptoms as they get sicker and sicker over time.

Chronic illness is in epidemic proportions. Despite the fact that the majority of the US population looks rather healthy, statistics show a different story. Nearly 1 in 2 (133 million) people have a chronic condition. This could be an illness like cancer or rheumatoid arthritis, or a condition such as arthritis, migraines or pain.[15]

"When the well's dry, we know the worth of water." —Benjamin Franklin, 1706–1790. When we are healthy we take it for granted. It's only when we get sick we realize the importance of good health.

The World Health Organization states, "Chronic diseases are diseases of long duration and generally slow progression. Chronic diseases, such as heart disease, stroke, cancer, chronic respiratory diseases and diabetes, are by far the leading cause of mortality in the world, representing 63 percent of all deaths. Out of the 36 million people who died from chronic disease in 2008, nine million were under 60.[16]

Your health or lack of it is based on your genetic vulnerability, the environment, and your lifestyle. Genetic variations are important but genes are like light switches that can be turned on or off based on the lifestyle you choose to live. The variations in genes, called

SNPs, are single nucleotide polymorphisms. SNP's can be tested for a person's ability to detoxify and for cardiovascular risk. This is important information so you can implement changes to decrease your risk of disease.

Seventy-five percent of gene expression is due to the environment or your lifestyle choices. Twenty-five percent is hardwired.

Sending you and your body parts off to multiple specialists may not be the best approach when many symptoms can be occurring that are linked to the same underlying cause such as inflammation. Maybe your doctor has mentioned that you have inflammation. In order for you to get well you need to find out the root cause of the inflammation. Treating your symptoms with an anti-inflammatory just covers the symptoms and may not be therapeutic.

Most physicians are not adequately trained to assess the underlying causes of complex, chronic disease and to apply strategies such as nutrition, diet, and exercise to both treat and prevent these illnesses in their patients. They practice more of an acute care approach; a quick diagnosis, followed by a prescription, procedure or surgery. This can be effective in management of acute medical conditions, but not necessarily the best answers for chronic conditions.

The vast majority of medical conferences and medical research are supported by pharmaceutical companies and biotech firms. Functional medicine courses, however, are often much more expensive to attend because they do not accept support from pharmaceutical companies or biotech firms, thus avoiding the potential bias in the information. Functional Medicine conferences have expert faculty found in clinical practices and university faculties. The education is delivered in non-biased evidenced-based presentations.

Seeing you as a whole person, eliminating the cause of the inflammation using specialized testing, and using effective natural therapies whenever possible is a functional medicine approach. Functional medicine addresses the underlying causes of disease, using a systems-oriented approach, and engaging both patient and practitioner in a therapeutic partnership.

The functional medicine physician looks at the whole person and partners with the patient. Functional medicine practitioners spend time with their patients, listening to their histories and looking at the interactions among genetic, environmental, and lifestyle factors that can influence long-term health and complex, chronic disease. The patient is treated as an individual and therapies are customized.

Despite advances in treating and preventing infectious disease, life threatening illnesses and trauma, this acute-care model is not effective in treating, healing and preventing chronic disease.

When no one knows what's making you sick, seek a physician who is trained in functional medicine to find the root cause of your symptoms or illness. There is an answer. You can and deserve to feel your best.

Sir William Osler, who is, perhaps, the most influential physician in recent history, once said, "One of the first duties of the physician is to educate the masses not to take medicine."[17] Individuals need to be encouraged to educate themselves and feel empowered to take positive actions to improve their health. And since we all have the power to heal ourselves, this is good news! Though drugs and/or surgery are sometimes exactly what we require, we can encourage our bodies to heal using natural approaches throughout treatment.

In many ancient Eastern traditions, the first key in the holistic healing arts is *awareness*—a relaxed focusing of the mind that is quite unifying and decidedly spirit-strengthening. A strong, bright spirit leads the healing process against disease so that we can fully grasp the nature of our current problems and have the energy to overcome them. Awareness practices that quiet the mind include silent contemplation, meditation, and self reflection; however, any relaxing or focusing experience where we pay attention such as appreciating nature or art, or playing a musical instrument can certainly bring peace to our minds.

Many times patients who come to me when asked what is causing their illness, they have the answer. Their intuition or insight has already provided some if not all the answers.

The second key in healing is *activity*. Certain activities blend with awareness practices very well including tai chi, yoga, and qi gong.

Other activities are equally important as well including sports, walking, gardening, weight training, or other exercise programs. In a survey of 22,000 physicians, it was discovered that 1 to 2 workouts per week reduced the risk of coronary artery disease (CAD) by 28 percent, 3 to 4 times a week decreased CAD by 34 percent, and more than 5 times a week, by 44 percent as reported in the *New England Journal of Medicine*.[18]

Furthermore, according to Eastern Asian healing arts, exercise builds digestive fire and therefore is necessary for us to receive the proper nutrients from our food. Without sufficient activity, we may find it difficult to make progress in health, regardless how nutritious our food may be.

With that said, key number three is *nutrition*. Dump your diet. Yes, you read that right. Dump your diet. This isn't about the numbers on a scale or a long list of shouldn't or couldn't. This is about YOU. It is about feeling FIT, STRONG and ALIVE. Turn back on sluggishness and lethargy and turn on self-confidence.

It's about radiance and a zest for life. It's getting back an abundance of energy. The right foods can ditch the doldrums. This is to look stunning, feel stunning, I've-never-felt-so-ALIVE lifestyle. This is about *finally* becoming who you were always meant to be: gorgeous, handsome, vibrant and UNSTOPPABLE.

You are going to love eating the right foods for you.

Coupled with exercise, nutrition represents a vital part of overall health and healing. The proper type of food and the quality of it, when digested thoroughly, benefits not only the biochemistry of our bodies, but also our brain function. It enhances the well-being of the mind, including how we feel and how we think.

High quality vitamins and minerals as well as proper supplements are essential for health. Your food choices should include colorful, fresh, whole fruits and vegetables. In particular, organic foods not only have fewer pesticides, 23 percent compared to 73 percent of conventionally grown foods, but in a study of 94,000 food samples from more than 20 crops, and they also contain more nutrients. Tests indicate that organic foods have substantially more minerals—as much as 90 percent compared to commercial foods.[19]

Furthermore, according to the *Journal of the American Medical Association*, just one serving per day of fruits and vegetables is associated with a 6 percent decrease in the risk of ischemic stroke (a result of insufficient, oxygen-rich blood supply to the heart).[20] And did you know that consuming cruciferous vegetables, such as broccoli, brussel sprouts, cabbage, asparagus, cauliflower, and spinach results in the prevention of potent cancers?

At Harbor UCLA Medical Center in Torrance, CA, a study was conducted to document the effects of broccoli consumption among men and women, ages 50 to 74. The results show that those who consume more broccoli (an average 3.7 half-cups per week) are 50 percent less likely to develop colorectal cancer than those who never eat broccoli.

Dairy has always been considered a good source of calcium and more often than not, we are still encouraged to "drink our milk" for healthy bones; however, numerous studies have shown that countries with the highest consumption of dairy also have the highest incidence of osteoporosis. *The Nurses' Health Study* found that those who consume the most dairy have the highest hip fracture rates. Dairy is often fortified with D2 (not a natural source) and then only in small amounts. One glass has about 100 International Units (IU). The recommended dose of Vitamin D is about 2,000 -5,000 IU depending on your Vitamin D3 lab results.

Vitamin D3, in its natural form (i.e. sunlight), is more effective than D2 and is important for bone maintenance and the absorption of calcium as well as contributing to the functioning of the reproductive system, the digestive system and the immune system. If the body does not have enough Vitamin D calcium is not well absorbed.

Most people do not spend enough time in the sun without sunscreen and their body exposed. As you age the skin is also not as efficient in converting the UV rays to vitamin D. If the body does not have enough Vitamin D, calcium is not well absorbed. Have your vitamin D3 level tested.

Rather than seeking the perfect nutritional plan that is instantly available and easy for all occasions, consider your current routine and how you might take steps improve it. Your well-being and ability to heal ultimately depends on taking time to care for your body, mind, and spirit and that includes proper nutrition.

Specific FDA approved labs are available to test your personal level of vitamins, minerals, fatty acids and amino acids. The results of these labs can then tell you and your physician where you are deficient. Then you, as an individual, can take the vitamins, minerals, minerals, fatty acids, amino acids, and supplements you need. Not any more or any less.

- Find a doctor that listens to you and can find the root causes of your illness or symptoms.
- Use specialized testing to make your best health choices.
- Enjoy your sacred time.
- Choose the activities that make your heart sing.
- Enjoy your food and the people you eat it with.

This year is a great year to bring balance into your life and bounce back into your step. A healthy mind, body, and spirit not only improve your health, but make your life more fun! Take the first step toward better health today.

Health is a choice. Always choose it.

Chapter 2

FOOD ALLERGIES:
DISCOVERY AND TREATMENT

He was not quite four years old and he had been sick since birth.

Chase was vomiting five times a day, had diarrhea three times a day, and suffered from severe asthma. He had nasal stuffiness, eczema, inflamed esophagus, acid reflux and difficulty sleeping. His parents had taken him to the pediatrician many times, the pediatric allergist many times, and the pediatric gastroenterologist many times.

He had not grown an inch or gained a pound in the last year. He was not able to attend pre-school because of his chronic illnesses. The treatment was pharmaceutical drugs, procedures, and surgeries. When I saw him he was on eight pharmaceutical drugs and had four surgical procedures.

The next recommendation was to operate on his stomach.

When I saw this darling little boy, my heart went out to him and to his parents who had suffered with him as they tried so hard to do the right thing. I tested him with one blood test checking for IgE food allergies and IgG (hidden) food sensitivities. He had many. Then, I tested him for gluten sensitivity—he was strongly responsive.

The family was educated in the planning of his new dietary needs, and within three days of avoiding the foods he was allergic and sensitive to, the vomiting and diarrhea stopped. His asthma and eczema have disappeared and he is now sleeping through the night. In six weeks he grew one and one half inches and gained two pounds. Within a year he grew 4 inches. He is off all medications and healthy.

Now he is an energetic healthy little boy who tells me he loves to swim and he is so good that he says he is "half fish and half human"!

A word from his mother…

Dr. Norling has truly been a life-saver to my four year old son, Chase. Prior to our visit, Chase had been suffering from multiple conditions; severe asthma, allergies, eosinophilic esophagitis, eczema and acid reflux. After many visits with multiple specialists, eight different daily medications and four surgical procedures, Chase was only getting worse. He wasn't thriving and didn't gain a pound or grow an inch for one full year. Luckily, we found Dr. Norling and right away she tested him to find out that he had severe food allergies and gluten sensitivities. She was also able to identify, through her extensive testing, that he had many different intestinal infections due to all the medications that were prescribed. Within three days of removing certain foods from his diet, his vomiting and diarrhea stopped. After only six weeks, Chase grew 1½ inches, gained two pounds, and is off all of his medications. He is now a happy, energetic and boisterous little four year old boy. He is perfect! I am so grateful to Dr. Norling for saving my son's life.

A word from Dr. Norling…

When his mother brought the lab reports to Chase's pediatrician and happily shared that Chase was well, the pediatrician glanced at the report and with a flip of his hand, dismissed it. Children, families, and patients deserve better. They deserve the right diagnosis and the right therapy.

Are the foods you are eating making you sick?

Do you have headaches, sinusitis, nasal stuffiness, heartburn, indigestion, irritable bowel syndrome (IBS), muscle aches and stiffness, joint pain, anxiety, depression, difficulty sleeping, fatigue, skin itching, inability to focus, palpitations, or mental confusion? You could have food allergies.

Many people suffer from food allergies or sensitivities and don't realize it. Rarely can we determine on our own that something we ate four days ago might be causing today's migraine. Many people needlessly endure years of illness and inflammation with numerous chronic illness and symptoms (arthritis, asthma, migraines, cluster headaches, bowel problems, irritability, eczema, hyperactivity, and many others) without even knowing that delayed food allergies may be causing these conditions.

"Food allergies," you say doubtingly.

There are two main food allergies; IgE (Immunoglobulin E) and IgG (Immunoglobulin G). IgE allergic reactions to foods can occur within minutes or a few hours after the food is eaten and may lead to many different symptoms including hives, swelling around the mouth, asthma, diarrhea, vomiting, and even life-threatening anaphylaxis (a severe adverse reaction involving the major body systems).

An antibody is a protein used by the immune system to identify and neutralize foreign objects like bacteria and viruses. Severe reactions to food allergies are most often caused by IgE, a naturally occurring antibody found in the lungs, skin and mucous membranes.

When the body produces too much of the antibody, it can create an immediate and severe allergic reaction triggered most commonly by consuming peanuts or shellfish. Though this affliction is rare, most people know when their body creates an abundance of IgE and are able to avoid the foods or allergens that could possibly trigger a dangerous allergic reaction.

Most people are aware of their IgE food allergies.

If the food eaten is a food allergen, the body will react like it is an invader. The immune system will attack it like it would a bacteria, virus, or parasite to protect your body. This creates inflammation. Inflammation is the underlying cause of illnesses.

Actual IgE food allergies are somewhat uncommon, with estimates that four percent of the population has food-based allergies. The most common food allergy triggers are the proteins in cow's milk, eggs, peanuts, wheat, soy, fish, shellfish, and tree nuts.

Some food allergies are more subtle. These types of food allergies (sometimes also referred to as a food sensitivity or intolerance), involve IgG antibodies and are measurable by an IgG food sensitivity test. IgG antibodies are associated with non-atopic, hidden, and delayed food reactions that can initiate, worsen, or contribute to inflammation and many different health problems.

These reactions are more difficult to notice since they can occur hours or even several days after consumption of an offending food. Often the offenders are frequently eaten foods that are hard to avoid, such as milk, corn, eggs, soy, and wheat. These could be your favorite foods! Every time you eat these foods, your immune system attacks it just like it would a bacteria or a virus trying to protect you from the offending food. Food allergies can create inflammation.

Symptoms and Diseases that may be Associated with IgG Food Sensitivities:

Fatigue	Dizziness
IBS	Recurrent infections
Heartburn (GERD)	Sinusitis
Headaches	Migraines
Sore throat	Muscle stiffness
Joint pain	Itchy skin
Mental changes	Sleep disturbances
Asthma	Arthritis
Canker sores	Depression

ADD and ADHD	Anxiety
Nasal congestion	Edema (Fluid retention)
Diarrhea	Constipation

Inflammation creates a multitude of symptoms and illnesses. It is the underlying cause of heart disease, cancer, diabetes, and Alzheimer's. These "hidden" food allergies are said to affect as many as 60 percent of the population.

Allergies and sensitivities to 90 different foods can be detected using just one blood test. But, more importantly, several studies have shown that avoidance of your food allergies leads to substantial reduction in the clinical symptoms mentioned in the previous table.

How does a patient acquire food allergies?

The tendency to be allergic to foods is either familial (genetic tendency) or by the constant and repeated exposure to the same foods. Since we tend to eat the same foods over and over, our present symptoms continue and new ones start to develop. Irritable Bowel Syndrome (IBS) or gastrointestinal inflammation can also put us at a higher risk for developing food allergies, and food allergies can cause IBS. A study published in *Gut* 2005, found that eliminating IgG food allergy antibodies may be effective in reducing IBS symptoms.[1]

Unfortunately, as we grow older and start to become pattern-eaters, we become sensitive to foods we always eat or crave. At a certain point, the body's immune system becomes overwhelmed by these foods and begins attacking weaknesses in the body.

The allergic food proteins are like foreign substances that the body is attempting to defend against. The manifestations are chronic conditions that over time become a chronic illness. The most damaging are the IgG and IgM antibodies that combine with serum protein and activate complementary reactions causing permanent cell damage; i.e. arthritis, multiple sclerosis, ulcerative colitis, Crohn's disease, and a whole host of other serious chronic conditions.

Both parents pass on the tendency to be allergic to certain foods. Normally, a small child will reject these foods in their diets. If at an early age we are forced to eat certain foods that we do not like or the foods disagree with us, then we tend to become allergic to these foods. Unfortunately, over time the food allergies create inflammation from repeated consumption which results in multiple chronic symptoms.

As improbable as it sounds, some people get symptoms from eating "healthy" foods such as wheat, milk, nuts, or even apples. For reasons we do not fully understand, sometimes eating a specific food causes the immune system to stand up and fight; yet the immune system loses. Consequently, you become ill. The illness you have is the immune system's allergic response to a certain food.

Food allergies create inflammation in the GI tract, and inflammation in the GI tract creates food allergies. Which comes first is the age-old question—like the chicken and the egg. What is known is that in order to effectively treat food allergies you also need to treat the inflammation in the GI tract. When treating the inflammation in the GI tract, you need to remove the food intolerances.

How can you find out if you're suffering from food allergies?

Skin tests, although fairly reliable for the detection of IgE foods allergies and environmental allergens, they are not well correlated with IgG food sensitivities, signs and symptoms. Elimination diets removing certain foods and then reintroducing them back into the diet give you some information. Placebo-controlled food challenges and elimination/challenge diets are time-consuming for the patient and require a high degree of patient motivation and compliance.

IgE and IgG food allergies or intolerances can easily be determined by testing 90–120 different foods with one blood test.

In the end, without testing, most doctors may not know what is causing your underlying problem so they will prescribe a medication for your symptoms. They haven't really cured the problem, but rather have hidden the symptoms so you can continue to function. Meanwhile, inflammation and other symptoms may surface and you will needlessly perpetuate your suffering. Most chronic diseases related to foods develop slowly, but become severe and resistant to routine treatment with medication. Unless the food is removed from the diet, the constant immune stimulation and inflammation persists.

Different treatment options are available—from over-the-counter products to prescription medications and allergy shots. While pharmaceutical medications are sometimes needed, there are both risks and benefits in using them. The action of medications is to block the body's natural response to an allergy. Antihistamines help block the action of histamine, a substance produced by our bodies during an allergic reaction which is a natural protective response.

Decongestants fight nasal congestion by constricting blood vessels. Prescription nasal steroids, or corticosteroids, are nasal inhalants that treat nasal allergy symptoms. If you believe the Nasonex® commercial, "There's no cure for nasal allergies, but there are Nasonex® treatments to help manage most symptoms," you would continue on the medication and eventually build a resistance to the drug.

The reality is if a hidden food allergy or sensitivity is causing the nasal stuffiness, elimination of the food resolves the nasal congestion. . If the nasal congestion is due to a fungal infection after many prescribed antibiotics, then this may need to be treated with herbs, a probiotic, or an antifungal. The right therapy is to find the underlying cause of the symptom rather than just treating the tip of the iceberg with a pharmaceutical drug.

The goal of immunotherapy (allergy shots) is to "train" your immune system over time to be better able to tolerate the allergens that trigger your symptoms. Other treatments include mast cell stabilizers, which help to prevent the release of inflammatory chemicals during an allergic reaction. The release of inflammatory chemicals is your body saying, "Help! What you are doing is not good for you!"

Symbicort®, a steroid used to help control asthma, contains *formoterol*, a long-acting beta$_2$-agonist (LABA). Medicines containing LABAs may increase the chance of asthma-related death. Medications may be needed, but it is always recommended to discover the underlying cause of the inflammation and remove it.

Your personal immune response system is what determines which foods give you symptoms. Hidden food allergies may be triggering your symptoms. The skin scratch test only tests the IgE and not the hidden IgG which is the cause of most of the inflammation. Make sure your doctor uses the right lab.

In addition to eliminating the food intolerances, vary the foods you eat each day. We all go to the grocery store with basically the same grocery list. We make the same 10–20 meals. We like them, they are a family favorite and they are "no-brainers". Eating the same foods can increase the risk of developing food allergies. Each food has its own micronutrients and macronutrients so eating a variety will give us more nutrients.

Are you suffering from hip pain? Stop eating eggs. Many times the hip pain is resolved.

I also recommend a multi-vitamin, B vitamins, magnesium, trace minerals, and essential fatty acids to my patients. Vitamin D is recommended depending on the lab results. Many times the patient is confused about "what should I take?" Sometimes the doctor is not sure.

For years I have clinically observed that when patients remove the foods they are allergic to, their environmental allergies or seasonal allergies also dissipate. Many common environmental allergies are linked to food reactivity or allergies.

Dr Gregory Plotnikoff, a good friend of mine and a highly respected colleague, lists common reactivities in his book, *Trust Your Gut*.

Common Allergy Reactivities (Plotnikoff)

Season	Environmental Allergies	Related Food Allergies
Spring	Birch pollen	Apples, carrots, celery, hazelnuts, peaches, pears, raw potatoes
Summer	Grasses	Tomatoes

Late summer	Ragweed Pollen	Bananas, melons, tomatoes
Fall	Mugwort	Apples, broccoli celery, some spices

Specialty tests that measure the level of nutrients in your body; vitamins, minerals, amino acids, and essential fatty acids are what I recommend. The results enable the patient and the doctor to know exactly what the patient needs. The recommendations can be specific. The patient is recommended specifically what they need, not anymore and not any less.

Gluten Sensitivity

Are you plagued by gastrointestinal (GI) symptoms? Are you afraid to go out to dinner because it could be your worst nightmare? The most obvious symptoms of intestinal permeability, also known as leaky gut, are the common symptoms such as bloating, cramping, constipation, and diarrhea.

Perhaps you are suffering from depression, brain fog, fatigue, poor muscle endurance or poor recovery from illnesses. You still may be experiencing autoimmunity, chronic inflammation, or other degenerative conditions after years of medical care. If these conditions are present it is very important to have proper laboratory testing. Intestinal permeability does *not* always have intestinal symptoms.

Many people are suffering from chronic inflammatory responses to their foods or diets. Gluten sensitivity and hidden food allergies are frequent causes of leaky gut. Other causes can be poor food choices, sugar, medications, stress, hormonal imbalances, neurological disorders, insomnia, and autoimmune disease (AI).

Type 1 diabetes has been associated with the triad of intestinal infection, intestinal permeability and an altered mucosal immune response. *Diabetes*, 2008, Oct; 57.

Leaky gut has also been associated with chronic heart failure, Inflammatory Bowel Syndrome (IBS) and obesity. If you have obesity, type 2 diabetes and insulin resistance you may want to have your doctor check your stool! I recommend using a specialty that checks the DNA. In the pediatric literature, leaky gut has been related to type 1 diabetes, allergies, asthma, and autism.

Clearly, intestinal permeability (leaky gut) has a major impact on your health. The first step is always finding the underlying cause of the disease or symptoms. Using specialty labs will give you the information you and your doctor need to create an individual plan for you.

Gluten sensitivity causes inflammation which can create intestinal permeability and both can cause autoimmune disease. There is no cure for autoimmune disease. Testing is critical. How can you prevent something or heal a condition if you do not know the underlying cause or issue?

Kevin, a 16 year boy, had been sick about three years. When he came to see me I was struck by what I saw. He was six feet three inches tall and weighed 100 pounds. He was suffering from severe stomach pains, lack of appetite, difficulty thinking and focusing, and fatigue. He missed months of school each year and was anxious and depressed.

He had seen his pediatrician many times and was told, "There is nothing really wrong with you." His doctor did, however, tell him and his mother that he had an eating disorder and was depressed. He recommended a mood-altering pharmaceutical drug and psychological therapy. His mother explained to the doctor that her son was depressed because he was so sick.

I did a comprehensive work-up and ordered specialty tests to determine any food allergies. The test was positive. I also checked for gluten sensitivity and it showed a strong reaction. I treated him with nutrient IVs and IV phosphatidylcholine. Within two months of discontinuing the foods he was reacting to, his stomach pains were gone, his mental function returned, his appetite was normal, and he gained 28 pounds. He was a happy teenage boy enjoying school. In this case, the right tests were done resulting in a right diagnosis and a list of the right foods for him.

My son Kevin, age 17, has had chronic stomach pains intermittently since kindergarten. We were able to manage the pains until Kevin entered high school. The stomach aches happened more frequently, and the pain became more severe. Kevin became depressed, withdrawn, and retreated into his room, refusing to go out with friends. Once a student with A's and B's turned into a student barely passing. He couldn't focus, concentrate, and became disinterested in school altogether.

We saw many doctors looking for answers to this ailment. One doctor thought it was teenage depression, which we ruled out with a psychiatrist. We saw a pediatric gastroenterologist, who called it IBS. We had no answers. Kevin missed about four weeks of school within a semester, and we were at our wits' end. A friend of the family, who had stomach ailments also, was seeing Dr. Norling, and recommended her to us. We went to see Dr. Norling, and after a few tests, Kevin was found to have food allergies to dairy and egg, and gluten sensitivity. His intestines were badly damaged. We eliminated those ingredients from his diet, and started him on a strict vitamin, mineral, and other medical supplement regimen.

Within a few months, the change was phenomenal. Kevin is once again, his smiling, bright eyed, rosy cheeked, happy self, earning A's and B's in school, socializing with his friends, and enjoying life. He reports that he has more energy, and is very happy that he is no longer sick. We are very thankful that we found Dr. Norling, and that she was able to give us the reason and cure for his ailment. We are grateful to have our son healthy once again.

Is gluten intolerance affecting your health?
Is your doctor testing for gluten sensitivity?

Do you have an auto-immune disease, a chronic illness or unresolved conditions? You may have gluten sensitivity or intestinal permeability (leaky gut). Leaky gut can be tested by Cyrex Array 2 lab. Intestinal permeability can lead to gluten sensitivity and gluten sensitivity can lead to intestinal permeability. Gluten sensitivity can develop antibodies which create tissue autoimmunity which has been shown to create auto-immune diseases. Perhaps you have tested for gluten and it came back negative. Many times the conventional labs are not comprehensive enough and report false negatives.

A comprehensive specialty lab (Cyrex Array 3) can now diagnose gluten sensitivity with accuracy.

Gluten sensitivity can occur at any age and is a major contributor to disease. The symptoms are both gastrointestinal and non-gastrointestinal. A simple blood test can stop the pain and suffering. In the past, there were many false negative reports on gluten sensitivity.

An estimated 20 percent of people have gluten intolerance, but only about five percent of the population knows it is the cause of their disease. There are estimates that gluten intolerance contributes to 300 illnesses. Here are just a few:

Diabetes, type 1	Brain fog
Autoimmune diseases	Hormonal imbalance
Thyroid disease	Infertility
Intestinal cancer	Anxiety
Intestinal lymphoma	Depression
Intestinal dysfunction	Liver disease
Fatigue	Rheumatoid arthritis

There is a direct relationship between gluten sensitivity and the development of auto-immune diseases (AID). Neurological disorders and impaired cognitive function can be directly related to gluten sensitivity. Before you blame your lack of focus and memory loss to stress or the menopause have a Cyrex Lab Array 3 blood test done to see if you are gluten sensitive.

Are you concerned you may be at risk for developing an autoimmune disease? Does hypothyroidism, diabetes and other autoimmune diseases run in your family? A specific test, Cyrex array 5, can identify antibodies already in your tissues *before* you develop the diseases. This is the silent phase of AI disease. The test can identify autoimmunity in the stomach, intestines, thyroid, adrenals, heart, reproductive organs, joints, bone, liver, pancreas and brain. Phospholipid antibodies can also be detected. If you are in the silent phase of AI there are things you can do to be in your best state of health.

If we wait until the conventional labs can identify autoimmune disease, there is already significant tissue damage. If we are looking to diagnose multiple sclerosis (MS) on a brain scan, there needs to be 70 percent demyelination (damage) in the brain before it can be detected. It makes much more sense to identify antibodies stuck to our tissue before we have significant tissue destruction. Then we can make life changes to help protect the tissue.

Celiac disease is an autoimmune condition determined by genetic markers of the small intestine, resulting in inflammation from gluten sensitivity that damages the lining of the small intestine. The damage is due to a reaction to eating gluten, which is found in wheat, barley, rye, and possibly oats.

About 5 percent of gluten sensitive patients have celiac disease. The treatment for gluten sensitivity and celiac disease is the same—avoid gluten. Period.

Celiac disease and gluten sensitivity can develop at any point in life—from infancy to late adulthood. The onset of illness most commonly occurs around age two, after wheat has been introduced into the diet, and in early adult life (third and fourth decades). People who have a family member with celiac disease are at greater risk for developing the disease. The disorder is most common in Caucasians and persons of European ancestry. Women are affected more often than men.

Specific screening studies show a much higher prevalence of 1:133 in the U. S. High risk groups for celiac disease include first degree relatives (15 percent) and individuals with type 1 diabetes and autoimmune thyroid disease. About 4–10 percent of patients with irritable bowel disease have celiac disease.[2]

Gluten Sensitivity and Leaky Gut

Most doctors don't specifically test for leaky gut. They typically rule out other disorders first and then consider whether the IBS symptoms meet the criteria for that condition and call it IBS.

That is where the mistaken diagnoses might come into play. Just because you have one symptom and not another doesn't mean that you do not have a gluten sensitivity.

Sadly, this is a very common problem. Researchers who have tested IBS patients for celiac disease have found between four percent and ten percent of those IBS patients actually have celiac, meaning a gluten-free diet should help to improve or eliminate their IBS symptoms.

It's also possible that some IBS patients who have been tested for Celiac disease and came up negative are gluten sensitive and will benefit from a gluten-free diet. Two recent studies have found that a one group of people with IBS, but without celiac disease, suffered from gluten sensitivity and saw their IBS symptoms improve or clear up when they eat gluten-free.

In the first study, researchers took 34 IBS patients whose IBS symptoms were controlled on a gluten-free diet and assigned 19 of them to eat gluten (two slices of bread and a muffin) every day for six weeks. The other 15 ate non-gluten-containing bread and muffins. After one week, those IBS patients eating the gluten foods reported significantly more pain, bloating, tiredness, constipation and diarrhea than the control group, indicating that the symptoms in this group of IBS sufferers were triggered at least in part by gluten.[3]

Another study conducted celiac disease genetic tests and a particular celiac blood test on people with IBS whose primary symptom was diarrhea, and then had them follow the gluten-free diet for six months. A total of 60 percent of those IBS patients who were positive for a celiac disease gene and in the blood test, plus 12 percent of those who didn't carry the gene and who received negative results on the blood test, found their IBS symptoms improved or resolved entirely on the gluten-free diet.[4]

If you've been diagnosed with irritable bowel syndrome but haven't been tested for celiac disease or gluten sensitivity, you should talk to your doctor about ordering these tests as well as food allergy tests.

Symptoms

The symptoms of celiac disease can vary with each individual. A review of celiac disease in the *New England Journal of Medicine* cataloged the myriad of diseases that can be caused by immune mitigated gluten sensitivity.[5] They can range from no symptoms at all to severe gas, bloating, diarrhea, and abdominal pain. Individuals suffering with celiac disease may experience severe symptoms such as diarrhea, weakness, and weight loss, indicating a marked decrease in the intestinal absorptive surface area involving much of the small intestine.

Experts comment that a thin person with type 1 diabetes is most often gluten sensitive. Individuals with hair loss are often gluten sensitive, too.

However, some individuals present with *anemia-related fatigue* and have gastrointestinal symptoms. With that said, symptoms do not always involve the digestive system. The disease can cause irritability, depression, generalized weakness, fatigue, and menstrual irregularities, just to name a few. The symptoms of celiac disease can also mimic those of other conditions such as irritable bowel syndrome, gastric ulcers, Crohn's disease, parasite infections, anemia, skin disorders, or a nervous condition.

Celiac disease and gluten sensitivity may also present itself in less obvious ways including irritability, depression or schizophrenia, stomach upset, joint pain, muscle cramps, skin rash, mouth sores, dental and bone disorders, and tingling in the legs and feet (neuropathy).

Dermatitis herpetiformis is an itchy, blistering skin disease that also stems from gluten intolerance. The rash usually occurs on the elbows, knees, and buttocks. Reactions to ingestion of gluten can be immediate, or delayed for weeks or even months. If untreated, malnutrition can occur. If left untreated too long it can be life-threatening.

Causes of Celiac Disease

Your small intestine is lined with tiny, hair-like projections called *villi*. Resembling the deep pile of a plush carpet on a microscopic scale, villi work to absorb vitamins, minerals and other nutrients from the food you eat. Celiac disease results in damage to the villi and without it, the inner surface of the small intestine becomes less like a plush carpet and more like a tile floor. As a result, your body is unable to digest and absorb nutrients necessary for optimum health and growth. Instead, nutrients such as fat, protein, vitamins and minerals are eliminated with your stool.

While the exact cause of celiac disease is unknown, the disease is often inherited. If someone in your family has it, there is a 10 to 20 percent chance that you may have it too. For reasons that remain unclear, many times the disease emerges after some form of trauma, such as an infection, a physical injury, pregnancy, severe stress, or surgery.

Screening and Diagnosis

Antibodies are specialized proteins that are part of your immune system and work to eliminate foreign substances in your body. In people with celiac disease, their immune systems may be recognizing gluten as a foreign substance and producing elevated levels of antibodies to destroy it.

In order to provide a proper diagnosis, the following tests are indicated:

- IgA human tissue transglutaminase (IgA-tTG): Occurs as an immune response to tissue transglutaminase and is rarely found in individuals without celiac disease.
- Serum IgA: Identifying serum IgA deficiencies are important for two reasons: First, IgA deficiencies can lead to false negatives for IgA-tTG. Second, individuals with an IgA deficiency have a 10 to 21 times greater risk of developing celiac disease.
- IgA antigliadin antibody (IgA-AGA): This antibody develops against gliadin showing consumption of gluten-containing foods that can cause celiac disease.
- To diagnose celiac disease a genetic marker, HLA DQ2, is positive in celiac disease 92–98% of the time. Another gene, HLA DQ8, is positive in 2–8% of celiac patients.
- The most comprehensive and accurate test is Cyrex lab Array 3.

Patients often come to me with a routine conventional lab showing the gluten test was negative. However, when retesting using Cyrex the patient was clearly gluten sensitive.

Use the most accurate test. Your life depends on it.

An intestinal biopsy can also diagnose celiac disease. The biopsy indicates if the villi which lines the intestines is damaged. The villi are important as they help absorb nutrients. When people with celiac disease eat foods or use products that contain gluten, their immune system reacts by damaging these villi. Malabsorption can occur no matter how much food is consumed.

Complications

Left untreated, celiac disease can lead to several complications:

- Malnutrition
- IBS
- Loss of calcium, magnesium, trace minerals and other nutrient deficiencies
- Osteoporosis
- Autoimmune diseases
- Lactose Intolerance
- Cancer
- Neurological Complications

People with celiac disease who don't maintain a gluten-free diet also have a greater chance of developing one of several forms of cancer, especially intestinal lymphoma and bowel cancer. People who are gluten sensitive and continue to eat gluten can increase their risk of colon cancer 40–100 percent.

Treatment of Celiac Disease

Treatment consists of a lifelong gluten-free diet. This sounds easier said than done as wheat is used as a filler and thickener in a number of prepackaged and restaurant prepared foods. Avoidance of gluten in the diet requires careful scrutiny of food labels for the presence of wheat and other offending grains such as rye, oats, and barley.

Products labeled wheat-free are not necessarily gluten-free. This includes any type of wheat (farina, graham flour, semolina, and durum), barley, rye, bulgur, Kamut, kasha, matzo meal, spelt, and triticale.

Amaranth, buckwheat, and quinoa are gluten-free as grown, but may be contaminated by other grains during harvesting and processing. Cyrex Labs Array 4 can identify cross-reactive foods. Then you will know what other foods and grains you may be able to substitute for the wheat.

Cross-contamination may also occur if gluten-free products are prepared in unwashed bowls previously containing gluten products. Oats may not be harmful for most people with celiac disease, but oat products are frequently contaminated with wheat, so it's best to avoid oats as well.

Cross-contamination may occur anywhere ingredients come together, such as a cutting board. You may also be exposed to gluten by using the same utensils as others, such as a bread knife, or by sharing the same condiment containers.

Individuals are encouraged to read labels carefully in order to avoid hidden sources of gluten which are found in soy sauce, all sauces modified food starch, ice cream, all soups, canned and frozen, beer, wine, vodka, whiskey, and malt. It is also found in most prepared and processed foods. Restaurant foods are often prepared or contaminated with gluten.

Gluten is found in ketchup, bran, imitation seafood, chewing gum, commercial salad dressing, sauces, salsa, artificial food colorings, canned vegetables, horseradish sauces, instant hot drinks—coffee, tea, hot chocolate; rice syrup, bouillon cubes, MSG, sausages, food stabilizers and the list goes on. In addition to wheat, other grains such as spelt, kamut, barley and oats contain gluten. Other foods can cross-react with gluten causing reactions.

Grains containing gluten are often used in food additives such as malt flavoring, modified food starch, and others. Other sources of gluten that might come as a surprise include medications and vitamins that use gluten as a binding agent, lipstick, postage stamps, and contamination of gluten-free foods with foods containing gluten.

When someone is diagnosed with gluten sensitivity, it affects everyone in the family. But, the main responsibility for keeping the individual healthy often falls on the mother or wife. To keep the kitchen clear of anything containing wheat, barley, rye, or oats may seem overwhelming and impossible.

The good news is many restaurants and bakeries have gluten-free choices. There are many foods you can eat—fresh fruits, fresh vegetables, high quality meats and fish, nuts, seeds, beans and depending on your food allergies, eggs and limited dairy may be options.

With the help of an experienced nutritionist, specialized cookbooks, support groups, and companies offering gluten-free foods and products, there *is* "light at the end of the tunnel." If you can't tell by the label if a food contains gluten, don't eat it until you check with the product's manufacturer. Look for gluten-free resources, recipes, and shopper's guide that can save you time at the market. Following a gluten-free diet may leave you challenged and frustrated at times and understandably so.

But the bottom line is such good news to find the root cause of your symptoms and be able to live a long and healthy life! The good news is there are many more options today.

With time, patience and a little creativity, you'll find there are many foods that you can still eat and enjoy. Be informed by the right resources—information can be empowering!

- Read food labels and call the manufacturer to learn more about the products you purchase.
- Seek out others with celiac disease for support, tips and recipes!
- If you're having difficulty coming up with suitable menus, talk to a knowledgeable nutritionist, search the internet for great recipes, stick to fruits, vegetables, lean meats, nuts and seeds, and healthy oils.

Just as a disclaimer; I do not have any financial interest with Cyrex labs. I recommend them based on their accuracy.

Chapter 3

INDIGESTION:
RIGHT TESTS RIGHT SOLUTIONS
FOR GERD AND IBS

A re you afraid to go out to dinner? When your friends call and say, "Let's go out for dinner," do you turn down the invitation knowing this could be your worst nightmare? Does your stomach feel like it is on fire? Do you need to be close to a bathroom when you eat?

If so, you just might have heartburn (GERD) or irritable bowel syndrome. The good news is that most digestive disorders are not diseases at all, but conditions which can be completely cured by finding the underlying causes of symptoms and removing the triggers.

GERD

Gastroesophageal reflux disease (GERD) is a condition in which the esophagus becomes irritated or inflamed. The esophagus is the tube stretching from the throat to the stomach. When food is swallowed, it travels down the esophagus to the stomach.

Symptoms include the following:

- Heartburn
- Reflux of bitter acid in the throat
- Hoarseness (especially in the morning)
- Feeling of tightness in the throat, as if a piece of food is stuck there
- Wheezing
- Bad breath
- Nausea
- Dental erosion

GERD affects nearly one third of the adult population in the United States to some degree at least once a month. Almost 10 percent of adults experience GERD weekly or daily. Even infants and children can have GERD.[1]

Factors that exacerbate the symptoms:

Lifestyle—use of alcohol or cigarettes, obesity, poor posture, stress.
Medications—including calcium channel blockers, aspirin, NSAIDS.
Diet—fatty and fried foods, chocolate, garlic and onions, drinks with caffeine, acidic foods such as citrus fruits and tomatoes, spicy foods.
Eating habits—eating large meals, eating too close to bedtime.
Other medical conditions—hiatal hernia, pregnancy, diabetes.

While these are contributing factors, the real question is, "What is the underlying cause of GERD?"

- Food Allergies
- H. Pylori infection
- Diet: Low fiber, high sugar, poor nutrients
- Medications
- Toxins
- Stress

Some would even say that it's not what you eat, but who you are eating with.

Hidden delayed immunoglobulin G (IgG) food allergies sometimes referred to as sensitivities or intolerances are often the cause of GERD. In my practice heartburn and reflux symptoms are related to food allergies and/or H.Pylori infection 95 percent of the time. Every time a person eats the food they are intolerant of or allergic to, the immune systems attacks it to protect the body and as a result, inflammation occurs. This inflammation is the body's natural response warning, "Something is wrong here."

The number of children with food allergies has risen 18 percent in the past decade according to a study recently published in the *New England Journal of Medicine*.[2] These food allergies can be identified by a simple blood test for sensitivities to 90 different foods. Once the food allergies have been determined and patients eliminate these foods from their diet, the esophagus and stomach begin to heal.

Natural anti-inflammatory food products containing medicinal properties such as glutamine, turmeric, ginger and other nutrients help the GI tract heal from the inflammation. Patients are often surprised that allergies to their favorite foods may be the culprit! They are also surprised and relieved at how quickly they began to feel better and when their heartburn, joint pain and itching have disappeared. They are surprised by the fact that they can comfortably stop taking Proton pump inhibitors (PPIs) even if they have used them for years. It is important to know that after the gastro-esophagus has been healed, the use of antacids or PPIs can be eliminated, *but this must be done slowly and gradually.*

Often when a patient sees a physician for GERD, the first therapy is an antacid or a PPI. These medications (over the counter or prescription) work by decreasing the acid in the stomach. *Stomach acid is there for a reason*—to digest the food you eat. If the acid is not there, the food becomes putrid and gas is created, which in turn irritates the esophagus.

When food enters the small bowel without having been adequately digested, the nutrients are not readily absorbed. The result is nutrient deficiencies.

Additionally, the acid serves to kill off any bacteria, viruses and parasites we ingest on a daily basis. Without the acid, a small bowel bacterial overgrowth

(SBBO) can then occur and contribute to the development of irritable bowel syndrome (IBS).

Antacid use has been shown to inhibit digestion of proteins and cause food allergies in animal studies.[3] "Stomach acid decreases with age, a condition called *hypochlorhydria*, which is related to the prevalence of atrophic gastritis in people over the age of 60. Hypochlorhydria (low stomach acid) is also associated with increased levels of Helicobacter pylori (H. pylori), an increase in proximal small intestine pH, small intestine bacterial growth, and deceased secretion of intrinsic factor, which is necessary for adequate absorption of vitamin B12."[4]

The use of antacids has multiple side effects and should not be used during pregnancy or by nursing mothers.

Many have interactions with other drugs. If necessary these should be used only for a short time until the underlying cause of GERD can be found and treated. The antacids and PPIs should then be tapered off under a physician's supervision.

The potential risks for users of antacids and PPIs according to *JAMA*, in 2004 are:[5]

1. Increased risk for infection
   - Bacterial overgrowth
   - C. difficle and Salmonella
   - Pneumonia
2. Malabsorption
   - Calcium
   - Iron
   - B12
   - Nutrients
3. Osteoporosis
4. Increased risk for food allergies
5. Stomach polyps
6. Acute nephritis (kidney inflammation)

Using antacids and /or having low stomach acid have been shown to initiate or exacerbate the following conditions:

- Asthma[6]
- Auto-Immune diseases such as Multiple Sclerosis
- Rosacea
- Gastric Cancer[7]
- Pernicious Anemia[8]

The side effects of all protein pump inhibitors (PPIs) include constipation, diarrhea, fatigue, headache, insomnia, muscle pain, nausea and vomiting. The following are some specific side effects for common PPIs:

Tagamet*
Major side effects include confusion and hallucinations (usually in elderly or critically ill patients), enlargement of the breasts, impotence (usually seen in patients on high doses for prolonged periods) and decreased white blood cell counts. Other side effects include irregular heartbeat, rash, visual changes, allergic reactions and hepatitis.

Pepcid*
Major side effects include agitation, anemia, confusion, depression, easy bruising or bleeding, hallucinations, hair loss, irregular heartbeat, rash, visual changes, nervousness, muscle pain, weakness, leg cramps, water retention and yellowing of the skin or eyes (jaundice).

Zantac*
Major side effects are rare. They include agitation, anemia, confusion, depression, easy bruising or bleeding, hallucinations, hair loss, irregular heartbeat, rash, visual changes and yellowing of the skin or eyes.

Nexium*
Nervousness, abnormal heartbeat, muscle pain, weakness, leg cramps and water retention.

Irritable Bowel Syndrome

Irritable bowel syndrome (IBS) is one of the most common disorders doctors see. IBS is not contagious, inherited or cancerous, but it is irritating! It's a functional disorder, meaning that the bowel doesn't work, or function, correctly. IBS often disrupts daily living activities.

Did you know that 70 percent of your immune system is located in your intestines? In fact, one of the primary roles of the gastrointestinal tract (GI) is to recognize and remove foreign molecules by using a complex, local immune system known as the Gut Associated Lymphoid Tissue (GALT). Because the intestines are essential to survival and are directly linked to the health of your immune system, it is important to know how to maintain proper functioning of your plumbing!

The immune system protects the body from infection, toxins, injury and food allergies (antigens). Though these afflictions can cause inflammation, it is the body's *normal* physiological response to injury. Chronic inflammation, on the other hand, is destructive and is responsible for a wide range of diseases. It is the ongoing presence of these inflammatory triggers that "fuels the fire" leading to chronic inflammatory diseases.

Intestinal permeability or "leaky gut" (characterized by large spaces between the cells of the gut wall that allow food, toxins and bacteria to leak out into your system) can be caused by food allergies, drugs, candida, parasites, intestinal bacteria overgrowth (dysbiosis) and enzyme deficiency. Leaky gut also increases the burden of liver detoxification.

The intestines are 25 to 30 feet in length with 100 square yards of surface area **(twice the length of a tennis court).** Over the course of a lifetime, the gastrointestinal tract processes 50–60 tons of food, chemicals and toxins. This material provides the building blocks for everything human. Imbalance in the GI tract affects every part of our body. Your GI tract can make you sick. Your GI tract can make you well. Nourish it, protect it and support it.

In a healthy intestinal tract, more than 98 percent of ingested food antigens are blocked from entering circulation. However, in a compromised environment with impaired digestion or increased intestinal permeability, significantly more food proteins (antigens) may penetrate through to the systemic circulation.

Remember the intestine is not a sewer pipe! It is a dynamic organ where absorption is highly organized, regulated and energy-dependent.

The number of bacteria in the large bowel is greater than 100 billion, which is more than the total number of cells in the human body. Intestinal bacteria produce toxins and anti-toxins, chemically alter food and drugs, produce and degrade vitamins, produce short-chain fatty acids from fiber, degrade dietary toxins and inhibit the growth of certain bacteria and pathogens. There are "good" bacteria, "bad" bacteria and candida or "yeast." But, it is important to realize that the general health of our intestines depends greatly on the *balance* of these substances throughout..

As many as one in five American adults have IBS, which begins before the age of 35 for 50 percent of people. Overall, about twice as many women have IBS. Twenty-five percent of people with GI infections will develop post-infectious IBS. IBS is a problem many people aren't comfortable talking about because the signs and symptoms may be embarrassing.

Signs of GI dysfunction
- Foul smelling stools
- Diarrhea/constipation
- Pain/cramping
- Nausea
- Mucus/blood in the stool
- Indigestion
- Excessive flatulence (gas)
- Bloating

Causes of IBS
"The causes of IBS include food allergies and infection including small bowel bacterial overgrowth (SBBO); 78 percent of IBS patients test positive for SBBO; 78 percent of fibromyalgia and 77 percent of chronic fatigue syndrome (CFS) patients have SBBO," according to research published in the *American Journal of Gastroenterology* in 2000.[9]

The cause of SBBO is slow transit time, low stomach acid or PPIs, maldigestion and lactose intolerance. Half of people over age 60 and 80 percent of people over age 80 have low stomach acid.

Stress plays a major role in the exacerbation of IBS by lowering the levels of serotonin, a calming happy neurotransmitter produced in the intestines. Low levels of serotonin can also cause constipation.

We used to think that neurotransmitters, "brain chemicals", were only produced in the brain. The gastrointestinal tract is not only 70 percent of our immune system, it digests our food, absorbs the nutrients and detoxifies, but it also produces neurotransmitters. It does that because it contains as many brain cells as the brain! We have always connected the two. One would say, "When I heard that, it made me sick to my stomach." Today through better research we know neurotransmitters are also produced in the GI tract.

Intestinal Bacterial Overgrowth and Pathogens

Equally important is the myriad of organisms that reside or invade the GI system. All too often, assessing intestinal bacteria (flora) is overlooked as a significant source of information concerning systemic or even local health problems. In the early 1900's, recognition that intestinal flora could have a major impact on health and disease was first popularized by the Russian Scientist, Eli Metchnikoff (1845–1916). He explored the idea of "dysbiosis," which he defined as a state of living with intestinal flora that may have harmful or detrimental effects. He said, "Death begins in the colon." He received the Nobel Prize in 1908 for his work.

This is hardly new news!

As more research is performed, the idea is now receiving significant scientific validation. In fact, mainstream medical journals including *Clinical Rheumatology, Archives of Internal Medicine, Journal of Clinical Gastroenterology, American Journal of Gastroenterology, Lancet, American Journal of Clinical Nutrition* and others have published research supporting the concept of dysbiosis (overgrowth of bacteria).

High-quality manufacturing of 'good' bacteria and all supplements is a must in healing. ConsumerLabs[10], an independent lab, recently tested 25 probiotic products. Eight products claimed a specific number of organisms per serving. Thirteen claimed only a number of organisms at the time of manufacturing, not the same number at serving. Eight out of the 25 products contained less than one percent of the claimed number of live bacteria or of the expected minimum of one billion.

The use of high-quality probiotics is essential; the range of therapeutic doses range from 15 billion species to 450 billion species. Research also shows that probiotics use decreases upper respiratory infections! *The European Journal of Clinical Nutrition*, showed that probiotics reduced the incidence of the common cold and shortened the days the person was symptomatic.[11] This makes perfect sense as 70 percent of the immune system is located in the gastrointestinal tract.

Always use good quality probiotics and supplements that are GMP certified or pharmaceutical grade. Don't waste your money or your health on products that are not going to give you the benefit you need. It is not a good investment.

Probiotics are not the same thing as prebiotics. Prebiotics are non-digestible food ingredients that selectively stimulate the growth and/or activity of beneficial microorganisms already in people's colons.

Gastrointestinal inflammation can result in a dramatically weakened immune system. We need the best immune system to protect us from cancer, bacteria, parasites, and viruses.

**Conditions directly associated with
or linked to GI dysbiosis or dysfunction:**

Acne	IBS
Eczema	Celiac disease
Psoriasis	Fibromyalgia
Fatigue	Food allergies
Gastritis	Migraines
Rheumatoid arthritis	Rosacea
Multiple chemical sensitivities	Intestinal bacterial overgrowth

Joint pain and stiffness	Chronic fatigue
Skin rashes	Memory loss
Abdominal pain	Recurrent infections
Brain fog	Failure to grow (children)
Immune dysfunction	Malabsorption

Stool tests should be comprehensive and accurate when testing for bacteria, H. Pylori, yeast, parasites, worms, digestive enzymes and anti-gliadin IgA, a gluten marker. The pH of the stool is strongly related to the bacterial release of pH-lowering organic acids and pH raising ammonia. The test should also determine how well the individual is digesting food and absorbing nutrients.

Routine stool tests are usually inaccurate. I recommend using a specialized comprehensive stool test from an FDA approved laboratory. It tests the DNA of the organisms. All bacteria, yeast, parasites, and worms have their own DNA making this test extremely accurate. How can we fix something if we don't know the cause? Have you had the right test?

Removing these organisms may require prescription or non-prescription medicines as a part of the healing therapy. The bottom line is that if your gut is not healthy, neither is the rest of your body. Taking antispasmodic or anti-diarrheal medications does not help IBS. They only mask the symptoms. Do the right thing.

Successful treatment of GI dysfunction includes:

The Five "Rs" to Remember when Healing Your Intestines and Improving Your Immune System:

1. **Removal:** Avoid foods you are allergic, sensitive or intolerant to. Treat intestinal dysbiosis and remove toxic exposure, hydrogenated / damaged, oxidized oils, sugar, fructose corn syrup, processed foods, sugar, gluten/grains. These need to be removed or at least minimized.

2. **Replace:** Replenish enzymes and other digestive factors including hydrochloric acid (HCl). Your doctor may suggest HCl to be taken at the start of meals that contain protein. The need for HCl is determined

by testing and also the clinically described symptoms of consuming meat and other concentrated protein that seem to just sit in the stomach and not move. This is particularly important if you are over the age of 60. Reduced HCl may impair the absorption of nutrients such as B12, folic acid, calcium and iron and may also predispose you to increased intestinal infections.

3. Many people experience nausea which is a clear sign of the gall bladder not releasing bile to digest fats and oils. Digestive support with bile salts may be necessary and required if the gall bladder has been surgically removed. As the food bolus moves from the stomach portion into the duodenum and beyond, bile salts as well as digestive enzymes and bicarbonate may be needed to help support the entire digestive process.

4. **Reinoculate:** Reintroduce the "good" bacteria or probiotics to establish a healthy balance of intestinal bacteria. Many over-the-counter probiotics may lack quality or may not contain a high enough dose. The probiotics should include Lactobacillus, Bifidobacteria, and Saccharomyces Boulardii especially when taking antibiotics. The addition of Butyrate, a short chain fatty acid, as a supplement sets the stage for the colonization of the friendly bacteria and is a critical piece in normalizing intestinal flora.

5. **Repair:** This is especially important when treating intestinal permeability. Repair refers to providing nutritional support for regeneration and healing of the gastrointestinal lining. Direct nutritional support is critical and must include balanced essential fatty acids (or hemp seed oil), phosphatidylcholine (only those brands with greater than 50 percent PC content), and EPA from fish oil.

    • Add GLA from Evening Primrose oil (Canadian source) along with butyrate, homemade/ bone marrow broth, aloe vera juice, balanced electrolyte concentrate, L-glutamine, N-acetyl-D-Glucosamine, and Vitamin B5—pantothenic acid.

    • Add zinc, mastic gum, bicarbonates (buffered C) if indicated by testing and fiber (ground flax seed, 100 percent flax crackers, seeds, nuts, asparagus, celery, green leafy veggies, etc).

- Medical food supplements are also a good support for repair of the GI tract.

6. **Rebalance**: Balance your hormones, your neurotransmitters, your foods, and your life! There is a dynamic dance between our gastrointestinal organisms, our environmental inputs, and the health of our immune system. Everyday we are getting a few little cancer cells in our body and lots of bugs from the environment which the immune fights off. Located in our GI tract our immune system is key to our health and our happiness.

Discuss with your healthcare professional regarding the right assessment and therapeutic options to treat intestinal dysfunction, imbalance or impairment. Healthy intestines relieve symptoms and conditions, make you feel better and support the overall health of your immune system!

Remember, your health starts in your gut!

- Test IgE and IgG food allergies and eliminate those foods.
- Test gluten sensitivity using specialized testing.
- Test for H. pylori using DNA lab.
- Get the right comprehensive stool analysis (absorption, digestion, inflammatory markers, bacteria, Candida and parasites).
- Test for intestinal permeability (leaky gut).
- Heal the GI tract by decreasing inflammation.
- See the right physician who can test for and recommend the five steps to treat GERD and IBS: *Remove, Replace, Reinoculate, Repair and Rebalance.*

You don't need to suffer. You can enjoy your food and the good times that come with it.

Chapter 4

HORMONES FOR LIFE:
HEALTH OR HARM?

Linda was 50 years old and perspiring! Embarrassed, she grabbed for her Kleenex in her already overstuffed purse. Not finding one she continued frantically searching to find one. Soon she was up to her elbows in her purse and I quickly came to her rescue with a tissue. She seemed frustrated and said, "I am continually irritated." She told a story about shopping the day before with her friend. "I told my friend, I had lost my thing. Her friend said, "What thing?" Linda told her, "My black thing." Her friend said, "What black thing?" Raising her voice Linda told her loudly, "You know the black thing I keep my stuff in!"

Linda then continued with her story. Her story consisted of memory loss, brain fog, stiffness, hot flashes, mood swings, difficulty sleeping and numerous menopausal symptoms. She had many questions about hormonal replacement therapy and bio-identical hormones.

As a board certified OB/GYN while full time faculty at the University of Minnesota Medical School in the Department of OB/GYN, I participated in numerous hormone research projects—including the Women's Health Initiative and the HERS study. This experience, together with advanced training in Bio-identical Hormonal Replacement Therapy (BHRT) for both women and men, gives me the confidence to know I can answer the questions and present the facts, not the fiction, surrounding the field of hormonal replacement today to help my patients make the best personal choice for themselves.

If I don't have the answer I research it. Women and men do not need to suffer from hormonal imbalances.

Susan is a bright 49 year old very successful business woman. This is her story.

> *"I came to Dr. Norling in, physically and mentally, the worst condition of my life. I had gained 38 lbs. on my normally thin frame, suffering from debilitating migraine headaches, fatigue, brain fog, depression, chronic constipation and bloating as well as diminished libido."*
>
> *"After repeated disappointment with countless physicians, specialists, and programs, Dr. Norling and the Mind Body Spirit Center have helped me achieve a renewed zest for life. I have an amazing sense of well-being and my migraines have been completely eradicated. I have returned to my normal healthy body weight and have boundless energy. Thanks to the personalized attention I received from Dr. Norling, I feel 20 years younger. Her diligent research and insight detected causes for my symptoms like allergies and metal poisoning when no other health care provider was able to do so. The program is a comprehensive one and provides everything needed to achieve optimum wellness."*
>
> *"I truly cannot say enough about my continued experience at the Mind Body Spirit Center. Dr. Norling and her staff have given me my life back."*

Are you one of the many women who are experiencing anxiety, depression, difficulty sleeping, pain, fatigue, brain fog, carbohydrate cravings, lack of motivation, muscle weakness, difficulty losing weight, hot flashes AND low libido? What used to be more, more, more, is now chore, chore, chore.

Or, maybe you are one of many men experiencing irritability, loss of energy, muscle wasting, increased body fat, osteoporosis, loss of libido, loss of an erection and depression? Maybe you are a woman who can identify with Suzanne Somers' Seven Dwarves in her newly released book, *I'm Too Young for This:*

1. Itchy
2. Bitchy
3. Sleepy
4. Sweaty
5. Bloated
6. Forgetful
7. All Dried Up

These symptoms are not a sign of growing older or just in your head. They are the result of hormonal imbalance and can occur at any age. They may be due to estrogen, progesterone, or testosterone deficiency—and yes, that includes men and women. They may also be due to low thyroid, an adrenal imbalance, or a neurotransmitter imbalance—neurotransmitters are the chemicals found mostly in the brain that effect all our moods, actions, and mental clarity.

One of the most important keys to your health and happiness is balancing your hormones. Hormones are in our body for good reasons. All of our moods, emotions, mental function, and physical health are affected by our hormone balance. All our hormones and neurotransmitters can and should be balanced. Remember, hormone balance not only includes the sex hormones of estrogen, progesterone and testosterone, but also thyroid, adrenal and neurotransmitter hormones. All these systems and hormones interact and support each other.

If you are experiencing any of the previously listed symptoms of hormone imbalance consider testing and seeing a physician trained and knowledgeable in this field who can treat you as an individual using natural effective approaches whenever possible. To get the best results and achieve optimum health, these systems must be tested and treated appropriately, using specific targeted natural amino acids, nutrients, and bio-identical hormone replacement therapy

(BHRT). BHRT is a natural effective hormone replacement without the side effects of typically prescribed pharmaceutical drugs.

One of the most complicated and difficult health care decisions menopausal and pre-menopausal women face today is whether or not they should use hormone replacement therapy (HRT). Do women and men need any hormones or natural remedies for this biological aging process?

Patients want to know if HRT is right for them, how they may benefit, how long they will have to undergo therapy to receive benefits, and if there are side effects or potential long-term risks.

No other pharmacologic drug has been as thoroughly studied as estrogen. The literature is vast and the messages are confusing. Many health care practitioners have a limited understanding of all the therapeutic options and the more global issues in menopause. So, how do you decide what is best for you during this transition?

First be clear that the Women's Health Initiative (WHI) used non-bio-identical synthetic hormones (Premarin and Provera)—in spite of the fact that there were positive findings. Today bio-identical hormonal replacement (BHRT) is often recommended for its effectiveness, fewer side effects, safety and natural approach.

USC published a review in *Cancer Journal* in 2009 noting that from 2002 to 2008, reports from the Women's Health Initiative (WHI)[1] claimed HRT significantly increased the risks of breast cancer development, cardiac events, Alzheimer's disease and stroke. The Women's Health Initiative (WHI) stunned and confused the nation and the medical community with the results that synthetic (HRT) posed more health risks than benefits.

Menopause and hormone imbalances are complicated matters.

These claims alarmed the public and health professionals alike, causing an almost immediate and sharp decline in the numbers of women receiving HRT.

However, the actual data in the published WHI articles reveal that the findings reported in press releases and interviews of the principal investigators were often *distorted, oversimplified, or wrong*. On these complicated matters, physicians and the public must be cautious about accepting "findings by press release" in determining whether to prescribe or take HRT.

What are the facts about the WHI Study?

The first fact is the design and methodology of the study was flawed. This was very unfortunate because women deserve to have the most accurate information to make the best personal choices for themselves. The *intent* was to determine the risks and benefits of HRT in normal healthy menopausal women. However, the WHI included women:

- 50 to 79 years old with a mean age of 63.
- 34.1 percent were overweight or obese.
- 49.9 percent were smokers.
- 3 percent had previous MI (myocardial infarction or heart attack).
- Women with hot flashes were excluded.

The women age 65–79 years old are at higher risk for CVD and cancer. Women 65–79 years of age generally are not on HRT. So the study took a high risk group that does not even take the hormones and pooled the data. In addition only the synthetic hormones, Premarin (estrogen) and Provera (progestin), were studied. The study did not include bioidentical hormones or crèmes. One fixed dose was used and not individualized dosing. The findings in the synthetic hormone WHI study were:

The findings for 12,304 women who took HRT for 5.3 years during the study were the following:

- No increase in breast cancer.
- No deaths in the breast cancer group.
- A 33 percent decrease in hip fractures.
- A 37 percent decrease in colon cancer.
- An increase in strokes and clotting but no increase in deaths.
- No increase in mortality from any cause.

The absolute numbers in 10,000 women there were 8 more breast cancers, 7 more heart attacks, and 8 more strokes in the group using HRT as compared to a placebo. Surprised? These are the facts.

One of the factors was all about age! According to Steven Goldstein, MD, professor of medicine at NYU Medical Center, "What we discovered is that if a woman is between the ages of 50 and 55 when she starts taking hormones, or if she begins HRT less than 10 years after she started menopause, she has less heart disease and less death from any cause, compared to the placebo group." These results were published in April 2007 in the *Journal American Medical Assoc.*[2] and then again reinforced by similar research published in *The New England Journal of Medicine* the following June.[3]

The WISDOM (Women's International Study of Long Duration Oestrogen after Menopause) study published in the *British Medical Journal*[4] duplicated many of the same findings detailed by WHI, **particularly concerning the increased risk of heart disease in older women who began or restarted hormone therapy long after menopause.**

The *Journal of Clinical Endocrinology Metabolism*[5] 2010 stated that data from various WHI studies, which involved women of average age 63, cannot be appropriately applied to calculate risks and benefits of HRT in women starting shortly after menopause.

The *Journal American Medical Association* in April 2011 concluded that out of 10,739 post-menopausal women in the WHI, with a prior hysterectomy who were treated with Premarin only for 5.9 years had a **lower risk** of breast cancer than women taking a placebo.[6] Additionally they were at lower risk than the placebo even when followed for another 5 years off the hormones.

No explanation was offered for this result. It now appears, however, that the breast cancer risk due to estrogens has been highly overestimated. It would also support the possibility that synthetic non-human identical progesterone, a progestin, which was not administered to the women who had a hysterectomy, maybe the responsible agent in prior studies revealing a greater risk of breast cancer in hormone-treated women.

In *Lancet Oncology* 2012, the use of estrogen alone for a median of 5.9 years was associated with *lower* incidence of invasive breast cancer, 151 cases, compared with placebo, 199 cases.[7] Harvard Nurses' Health Study published in the *Archives of Internal Medicine* reported that those women who took estrogen only experienced an increase in breast cancer after 20 years of use according to Cynthia Stuenkel, MD, professor of medicine at the University of California at San Diego.[8]

The question now being raised by researchers and clinicians is, are the risks increased by the synthetic progestins? All studies using oral synthetic HRT have shown an increase in strokes and gallbladder disease. But there is lack of consistent data.

According to the Mayo Clinic, the WHI data analysis revealed that participants aged 50 to 59 who took estrogen only experienced **fewer** heart attacks and deaths from coronary heart disease with a 50 percent decrease in cardiovascular disease. There were fewer cases of invasive breast cancer than the participants who took the placebo![9]

Oral synthetic HRT have shown an increase in strokes and gallbladder disease. There is also an increased risk of uterine cancer when unopposed estrogen is used in women who have not had a hysterectomy. Women who have a uterus need to use Progesterone to protect their uterus if they are using estrogen.

We know that HRT decreases the risks of osteoporosis, colon cancer, menopausal symptoms, and supports mental function. But what about sex?

Sexual activity at baseline in the WHI was 60.7 percent age 50–59, 44.9 percent, age 60–69 and 28.2 percent in 70–79 year olds. Most of the participants were satisfied with their current sexual activity (63.2 percent). *Of those dissatisfied, 57 percent of the women preferred more sexual activity.* HRT was associated with a higher percentage of participants reporting sexual activity.

Additional benefits:

Recent studies have also shown a decrease in short-term memory loss and a reduction in diabetes risk by 12 to 21 percent. A 2004 study published in the *Journal of Alzheimer's Disease (AD)* showed HRT had favorable mental effects across multiple cognitive areas, including memory and visual memory in postmenopausal women with AD.[10]

Bio-Identical Hormones (BHRT)

Are natural therapies better for treating menopausal symptoms? Do women need any hormones or natural remedies for this biological aging process? Synthetic HRT is associated with benefits and risks. What about BHRT?

The literature is vast and the messages are sometimes confusing. Let me try to help decipher this information for you.

Synthetic hormones are derived from plant progesterone and animal estrogens, but are not identical to the hormones your body uses (generally an extra covalent bond or molecule is added so that it can be patented). Synthetic hormones act as toxins because their chemical makeup cannot be metabolized properly. The synthetic pharmaceutical drugs such as Premarin, Provera, and Prempro can be patented.

Bio-identical hormones are made in the lab and have a chemical structure that is identical to the hormones made by your body. Because they are natural they cannot be patented.

Compounded bio-identical hormones may be your best option. In this approach the physician may use specialized testing to measure your existing hormone levels. Based on the results, your physician can then prescribe a hormone supplement for you that may include several hormones matched to your individual needs.

BHRT compounded estrogens are generally used in lower doses owing to the combined effect of the weaker estriol along with estradiol. These natural estrogens are thought to be metabolized significantly differently by the body, have a shorter half life, and can be used in customized dosing regimens and potencies to fit each individual woman and clinical situation. They can be adjusted to be stronger or weaker in small amounts to taper someone on or off of hormones.

Customization through a compounding pharmacy can maximize the therapeutic effects while minimizing the potential for adverse effects. The quality of a finished compounded drug product can be affected by many factors, including the quality of the active pharmaceutical ingredient, the compounding practices of the pharmacy and training of the compounding pharmacists.

Choosing a reputable experienced compounding pharmacy is crucial. Choosing a reputable experienced BHRT doctor is crucial.

Estradiol, progesterone and testosterone are FDA approved. Progesterone is the only bio-identical hormone available over the counter (OTC) but there is a wide range of quality in this low dose progesterone and OTC products are not recommended. The FDA requires manufacturers of FDA-approved products that contain estrogen and progesterone to include a black box warning about the risks. However, compounded products are exempt from providing patient package inserts that contain warnings and contraindications for estrogen and progesterone.

According to the Mayo Clinic, "there is no evidence that bio-identical hormones are safer or more effective than standard hormonal replacement therapy."[11] However, new research has been published showing the increased safety using BHRT.

Estriol, most often the predominate estrogen in BHRT has *not* been associated with an increase risk of breast cancer, *International Journal of Cancer.*[12] The transdermal estriol was also *not* associated with an increase risk of uterine cancer, *Menopause.*[13] Estriol has been shown to increase bone mass, improve urinary incontinence and vaginal atrophy. Natural progesterone crème has been correlated with a decrease risk of breast cancer and supports cardiovascular health. It also is calming, supports sleep, increases metabolic rates, and is a natural diuretic.

According to the Centers for Disease Control and Prevention (CDC), heart disease is the leading cause of death in women. Menopause can cause elevations in blood pressure, LDL cholesterol, total cholesterol, triglycerides, as well as homocysteine levels, C-Reactive protein, and interleukin-6, **which are all related to estrogen deficiency.**

Multiple other research articles published in mainstream medical journals by Shairer, Espie, Dew, Saeki, and Batur all found no increase in breast cancer using BHRT and many find a negative correlation. This is all good news. Women are comfortable in choosing the option of BHRT when there is research showing the effectiveness and safety.

In considering hormones, don't forget testosterone. Testosterone is a female hormone which not only increases sexual interests, but increases the sense of well-being and muscle strength. It helps to maintain memory, keeps skin from sagging, helps maintain bone health, and decreases excess body fat.

Continued research must be done on BHRT to study the clinical outcomes and long term effects.

Getting Started

I highly recommend women obtain 2-OHE1 and 16-OHE1 estrogen levels before and after taking estrogen. This test determines how you are metabolizing estrogen and may help you and your doctor identify if you are at a higher risk for developing breast or other cancers. Estrogen is metabolized by two pathways; the 16-OHE1 may increase your risk of cancer and the 2-OHE1 is protective against breast cancer.

The good news is that it is possible to change the pathway in favor of the protective 2-OHE1 by eating cruciferous vegetables (e.g., broccoli, brussel sprouts, cabbage and cauliflower), soy and omega-3. Nutritional supplements containing Indole-3-carbinol (I-3-C) or DIM also support the 2-OHE1 metabolism. Iodine supplementation has been shown to change the pathway to the safer 2-OHE1.

Feeling your best usually takes more than just the right prescription. Consider trying the most natural, least invasive steps first to create a foundation of health and hormonal balance, gradually adding remedies if and when they are needed.

Balanced hormones are the key to health and every person is unique. As hormones decline, health declines and aging accelerates. Decisions about whether to start, stop or change your hormones should be made on an individual basis only after consulting your physician and a knowledgeable pharmacist. Whatever choices you make when deciding your course of action, should be taken seriously with accurate and balanced information.

Christiane Northrup's, *The Wisdom of Menopause*, 2012 is a wealth of information for women and men.

A scientific advisory panel to the American Menopausal Society issued a position statement on hormones in *Menopause*, March 2007. Panel chair Wulf

Utian, MD, PhD, of Case Western Reserve University states, "For women with severe menopausal symptoms, within a few years of their last period, hormone therapy shouldn't be as scary as it has been made out to be."[14]

The average age of menopause is 51, ranging from 40 to 58 years. Interestingly, after menopause the ovaries can continue to produce small amounts of estradiol, as do the secondary hormone-producing sites, such as the adrenal gland and fat cells. Consequently, it is not likely, but biologically possible for a woman to produce enough of her own estrogen to support her health throughout the second half of her life.

Menopause can, however, create dramatic physical and emotional changes, which create memories that remain with a woman throughout her lifetime. It is important to note that menopausal therapies include not only hormones, but mind, body, and spirit support.

I recommend a solid foundation that includes but not limited to:

- Choosing a knowledgeable experience BHRT physician that listens to your story. www.ForeverHealth.com
- Being your own advocate and participate in the decision making process.
- Getting the right testing.
- Using BHRT
- Choosing a reputable compounding pharmacy that specializes in compounding products rather than using a general pharmacy.
- Balancing all of your hormones.
- Using the optimal dose of hormones and only what you need in high quality supplements.
- Avoiding caffeine and smoking.
- Avoiding processed foods and sugar.
- Eating six, small, healthy meals per day with lots of fresh fruits and vegetables.
- Taking multivitamins and minerals, and essential fatty acids.
- Exercising consistently.
- Being good to yourself.

The primary purpose is to manage the transitions, prolong life and preserve a healthy, active lifestyle. The approach to achieving these important goals is to *normalize* as many hormones as possible by using natural approaches.

Be informed. The choice is yours. But remember—laughter is the best medicine.

Hormones for Women and Men

Recent research shows that low testosterone can increase the risk for cardiovascular disease (CVD), insulin resistance and increased mortality from CVD and cancer.

Hormones are in our body for good reasons. All of your moods, emotions, mental function, and physical health are affected by your hormone balance. Hormone balance must include the sex hormones of estrogen, progesterone and testosterone but also thyroid, adrenal and neurotransmitter hormones. All these systems and hormones interact and support each other.

Frequently pharmaceutical drugs are prescribed for mood disorders without testing resulting in less than satisfactory results and many side effects. The side effects are too many to list here but include sedation, lack of coordination, impaired memory and cognition, sexual dysfunction and, after chronic use, physiological dependence and the potential for addiction.

These drugs are often prescribed without even testing the neurotransmitters or other hormones. Nationally certified and highly respected labs are available to do specialized neurotransmitter testing. Menopausal symptoms may be due to nutrient deficiencies, low blood sugar, hormonal or neurotransmitter imbalances.

Hormones and neurotransmitters can be balanced without using drugs.

What about erectile dysfunction and men's hormones?

A study reported in the *Journal of Sexual Medicine* (Vol. 10, Issue 2, 2013) quantifies the cost burden of testosterone deficiency in men. Scientist examined 6 national databases and found testosterone deficiency was affecting 13.4 percent of men between the ages of 45 and 74. They also estimated low testosterone was involved in approximately 1.3 million new cases of cardiovascular diseases, 1.1 million new cases of diabetes, and more than

600,000 osteoporosis related fractures in the first year it is present. This results in up to $525 billion in healthcare expenditures in the U.S.

All men should be tested for low testosterone. It is a public health issue and your life depends on it.

Examining Erectile Dysfunction's Causes & Cures

Bob came into my office like many other men—his wife made him come. Bob was "just not himself." Previously they had enjoyed a frequent fulfilling sex life. Over the last year Bob seemed less interested, more tired, and had difficulty having an erection. He had been prescribed Viagra but it was not as effective as both of them would have liked. Bob was in good health but he had never had his testosterone checked. I ordered the lab tests for him and the results were 250 ng/dl, which is below the normal range.

After evaluating for other causes that may have been contributing to Bob's symptoms, it was clear his symptoms were due to "Low T." Bob was placed on bio-identical testosterone and the following month he cheerfully reported he was feeling like an18 year old and he and his wife were going on their second honeymoon!

Low testosterone also has significant health risks. Multiple mainstream medical journals have shown the dangers of low testosterone. Testosterone below 250ng/dl increases the all-cause mortality by 2.32 times![15] The cardiovascular mortality is also more than doubled to 2.56 times the risk. Cancer mortality is more than tripled at 3.46 times the risk. So men, for your health and well-being, have your testosterone levels checked and seek the appropriate treatment. Your health and happiness depends on it.

If you have difficulty achieving or maintaining an erection, you may want to take a look inside your medicine cabinet. There are a number of prescription and over-the-counter drugs that may lead to erectile dysfunction (ED). While these medications may be prescribed to treat a disease or condition, they could unsuspectingly be affecting your hormones, nerves, or blood circulation, resulting in or increasing the risk of ED. Medications account for 25 percent of ED.

Impotence, or ED, is the inability to achieve or maintain an erection more than 20 percent of the time. Erectile dysfunction affects 18 to 30 million men and can affect all age groups. This number has increased significantly as awareness of the disorder has heightened and more prescriptions are written.

ED is one of the most common sexual problems and affects nearly 50 percent of all men over the age of 40 at some point. In the past it was commonly believed that ED was caused by psychological problems; it is now known that 80 to 90 percent of impotence is caused by physical problems.

There are risk factors for the development of ED. As men age, the level of circulating testosterone decreases. This may interfere with normal erection. Low levels of sexual desire, lack of energy, mood disturbances, and depression can all be symptoms of low testosterone. Low levels of testosterone also can cause muscle wasting and decreased strength. Men might note they are shaving less or experiencing hot flashes, sweats or fatigue.

By far, the most important cause of the development of ED is the presence of illnesses like high blood pressure, diabetes, high cholesterol levels, and cardiovascular disease. Diabetes can be the cause of ED in more than 50 percent of men (three times as high as in non-diabetic men). These conditions, over time, can lead to a degeneration of the penile blood vessels.

Common causes of erectile dysfunction include the following:

- Prescription drugs
- Heart disease
- Vascular disease
- High blood pressure
- Diabetes
- Obesity
- Metabolic syndrome
- Hormonal imbalance (low testosterone)
- Advancing age
- Chronic illness
- Surgery or trauma
- Anxiety and depression
- Fatigue
- Poor communication or conflict with your partner

A vicious cycle often plays out in our society. Over 200 commonly prescribed drugs are known to cause or contribute to impotence. Poor lifestyle choices which lead to illness can also cause ED. Further, the drugs used to treat these illnesses can cause ED. But too often the drugs used to treat the resulting ED should not be used to treat the original illnesses, nor should they be combined with the drugs that caused the ED in the first place.

Drugs affecting impotence include the following:

- Anti-hypertensives
- Statins
- Anti-depressants
- Anti-anxiety drugs
- Antacids used to treat heartburn, acid indigestion, and GERD
- Diuretics
- Non-steroidal anti-inflammatory drugs
- Prostate cancer medications
- Medications to treat benign enlargement of the prostate
- Parkinson's disease medications
- Anti-arrhythmia drugs
- Muscle relaxants
- Anti-epileptic drugs
- Chemotherapy drugs

The best rule of thumb is to consult your doctor before modifying or discontinuing any prescription drugs.

There are only three oral drugs approved by the FDA to treat erectile dysfunction: Cialis, Levitra, and Viagra. All work by increasing the flow of blood into the penis so that when a man is sexually stimulated, he can get an erection.

There are certain situations in which these drugs may not be safe to take. If you have suffered from a heart attack, stroke, or life-threatening arrhythmia (irregular heart rate) within the last six months, you should discuss other options with your doctor. It is also advised to avoid these drugs if you have uncontrolled high or low blood pressure or if you experience chest pain during sexual activity.

Side effects of these drugs can include:

- Headache
- Upset stomach or "heartburn"
- Flushing (feeling warm)
- Nasal congestion
- Changes in vision (color, glare)
- Back pain (with Cialis)

Stop taking these medications and call your doctor or seek emergency medical treatment immediately if you experience any of the following:

- Rash
- Painful erection
- Prolonged erection (longer than four hours)—Most men would just think this was an answer to a prayer
- Fainting
- Chest pain
- Itching or burning during urination
- Sudden or decreased vision loss in one or both eyes (NAION, non-arteritic anterior ischemic optic neuropathy)

NAION causes a sudden loss of eyesight because blood flow is blocked to the optic nerve. On May 27, 2005 the FDA confirmed it was investigating a possible relationship between the use of Viagra and NAION.[16] This was originally noted by Dr. Howard Pomeranz, an eye expert at the University of Minnesota in 2000. Since then, there have been several other similar reports. In a study in the *Journal of Neuro-Opthalmology*, Dr. Pomeranz noted seven new cases of NAION in men taking Viagra. Pfizer has issued a press release saying it has found no link between NAION and Viagra.[17] People who have a higher chance for NAION include those who:

- Are over 50 years old
- Smoke
- Have heart disease
- Have diabetes
- Have high blood pressure
- Have high cholesterol

The recurring cycle of disease, prescriptions, and adverse reactions can be prevented in almost all cases by finding the underlying cause of the illness and addressing it with a therapeutic lifestyle program. Is the high cholesterol due to food choices, lack of exercise or low thyroid? Is it a genetic variant which can be tested? Will specific effective heart-healthy supplements such as CoQ10, garlic, omega-3 fatty acids, niacin, or red rice yeast lower the cholesterol? Is the high blood pressure due to low levels of Vitamin D or high levels of nor-epinephrine?

What are the stress factors? Are carbohydrate cravings that elevate the blood sugar a result of low levels of serotonin and/or poor food choices? Is the individual supported in a program that is scientifically based and provides education on nutrition, exercise, stress management and appropriate supplements to help maintain normal blood sugar and healthy weight loss? Is a neurotransmitter imbalance contributing to your ED?

Lifestyle choices can lead to degeneration of the erectile tissue and the development of ED. One way to improve ED is to make some simple lifestyle changes. For some men, adopting a healthier lifestyle such as exercising regularly, eating a healthy diet, and reducing stress may be all that is needed to find relief.

Poor dietary choices may lead to vascular disease (the most common cause of ED), which interferes with the erection process by restricting blood flow to the penis. Vascular disease (atherosclerosis) accounts for 50 to 60 percent of ED in men over age 60.

Smoking, drug or alcohol abuse will compromise the blood vessels of the penis. Lack of exercise and a sedentary lifestyle will contribute to the development of ED. Lean and physically active men are less likely to have problems with ED.

Seek a professional to guide you through the myriad of effective natural therapies, including acupuncture, herbs, and homeopathic remedies. Also keep in mind that good nutrition can support erectile function by improving overall health.

For those who require more intensive treatment, adopting these lifestyle changes in addition to other treatments can help.

Successful management of ED includes the following:

- Identify the underlying causes of health issues.
- Get hormonal testing—total and free testosterone.
- Seek natural approaches to attain optimal health.
- Make therapeutic lifestyle changes.
- Quit smoking, avoid excessive alcohol and drug abuse.
- Reduce stress and anxiety.

Recently, I heard Dr. Abraham Morgentaler, Associate Clinical Professor Harvard Medical School speak at a national conference. According to him, low T is incredibly common. Testosterone declines as men age. In my practice I have seen men in their early 40's with low testosterone.

Men with low testosterone often experience decreased sexual desires, erectile dysfunction, and difficulty achieving orgasm.

There are multiple other symptoms that are sexual in nature that also occur. Men experience fatigue, lack of motivation, mood changes and depression. Is your spark missing? Women tell me, "My husband is so crabby. He never used to be like that."

This is not just a sign of aging but it is often a sign of a hormonal deficiency.

Physically, men experience a loss in strength and less muscle tone. This is coupled with increased weight and an accumulation of abdominal fat. Serious health problems can also occur. One third of men with diabetes have low testosterone. Men can also have anemia and bone loss and approximately 20 percent have osteoporosis. The percentage is most likely higher because men do not often get a bone mineral density test done which diagnoses osteopenia or osteoporosis. Recent research also indicates that low-T in men increase the rate of cancer 3.5 times and more than doubles the risk of cardiovascular disease.

Low T is strongly associated with:

- Abdominal obesity
- Elevated fasting blood sugar
- Insulin resistance
- Abnormal lipids
- High blood pressure

According to studies by James, TH in *Diabetes Care,* 2011 testosterone therapy improves metabolic syndrome.

Once your labs have documented the level of your low testosterone you can be treated with injections or bio-identical testosterone crèmes. Pharmaceutical gels are also available but I recommend the bio-identical crèmes.

How do men feel when their hormones are balanced and their low testosterone has been treated to the point that it is a normal level?

1. "I feel like myself again"
2. "I feel normal"
3. "My wife enjoys spending time with me again"
4. "I have more patience with my children"
5. "I don't have to plan for sex like I did with the pills"
6. "I feel younger"
7. "I wake up with excitement for my day"
8. "I have taken that my hobby again"
9. "I feel alive"

Why don't all physicians caring for men test testosterone levels?

As men age the testosterone lowers and prostate cancer increases. For many years there has been a fear that testosterone may increase the risk of prostate cancer. However, there are many main stream medical journal articles that now show that this may be a long held myth by the medical profession.

In a recent article in the *Journal of the National Cancer Institute* 2008 the authors of eighteen separate studies from around the world pooled their data regarding the likelihood of developing prostate cancer based on concentrations of hormones, including testosterone. This was a large study which included more than 3,000 men with prostate cancer and more than 6,000 men without prostate cancer.[18]

No relationship was found between prostate cancer and any hormones studied, including total testosterone, free testosterone, or other minor androgens. In the accompanying editorial, Dr. William Carpenter and colleagues from the University of the North Carolina School of Public Health also suggested that scientists finally move beyond the long-believed [but unsupported] view that high-T is a risk for prostate cancer.

Recently, physicians have begun recommending that men stop getting routine PSA screening tests for prostate cancer, or at least get them less frequently, since an elevated PSA may indicate the presence of a disease but also may be the result of inflammation, infections, or simply riding a bicycle. Even when the cancer is real, in many cases it grows so slow that, as doctors say, the patient would have died with it, not of it.

For every 1,000 men in the 55–70 year old age group who undergo annual PSA testing over the course of 10 years, a single life will be saved. Meantime, up to 200 will undergo a biopsy, and up to 100 will have their prostate removed unnecessarily.

So is your doctor wrong or just not current with the literature?

Doctors in busy practices often don't have the time or take the time to read their own literature. We all need to be our own advocates. The good news is there are many effective therapies for ED and low testosterone. Explore your options. Put zest back into your life and a bounce back in your step.

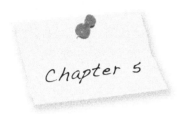

Chapter 5

SEX: WOMEN WANT MORE

D o you want to live longer? Then supercharge your sex life.

You have the opportunity to totally redefine your sex life. If you are an empty nester, you don't have to worry about kids at home. You may have an empty bed that you can fill with whomever you want. Here is a chance to redefine who you are as a sexual being—and we all have that chance.

The world of human sexuality is dramatized by reality television and affected by advertising. The media, celebrities and pop culture define a very specific look as "sexy." Women's round hips and big breasts are desirable, while other physical traits are not. However, the attributes that are supposed to be universally desired are, in fact, not universal at all. Beauty is defined differently according to culture and time period. The one steadfast commonality is that we are most truly aroused by the individual within our partners.

Perhaps we have lost sight of the meaning of a healthy sexual relationship with a partner. Maybe we don't find ourselves "sexy" compared to 120 lb. models in lingerie commercials, magazines and on reality T.V. shows.

You don't have to believe the story of your lives that you have been told. You're not the same person you were when you first had sex and not the same person today that you're going to be five years from now. There's always the opportunity to reinvent yourself, rediscover yourself, rejuvenate yourself, and redefine who you want to be as a sensual sexual person. All it requires is the courage to be fearless, to open your heart, to let go of the judgments you've internalized. Now is your time.

Where is the sex?

For whatever reason, has sex lost its appeal? What used to be more, more, more is now chore, chore, chore. What if a partner's physical attributes don't stimulate us? What if the mind is there but the body isn't? The only thing you want to do in the bedroom these days is pull the covers over your head and hope your partner doesn't get frisky.

What's going on? The problem could be inhibited sexual desire, defined by doctors as a lack of interest in sex or an inability to become sexually aroused. The possible causes vary greatly. Sometimes there is an obvious reason, such a hormone deficiency or depression.

It may be due to a health-related problem, fatigue, decreased energy, sleep disturbances, PMS or headaches. Often there is a hidden problem such as excessive stress, trouble in your current relationship or past abuse, all of which have significant impacts on sexual intimacy. These problems may need to be treated or resolved before you experience a change in your libido.

Libido and subsequent sexual activity is a mind, body and spirit phenomenon. A woman is more sexually receptive and thinks it is "sexier" if her husband or partner helps with the dishes than if he or she brings home a bouquet of fresh flowers.

In today's busy world, exhaustion and burnout leave many women with little energy left for the intimate lives they desire. Parents who partner in child rearing and household activities often have more satisfying sexual lives. A woman, who has a good relationship with her sexual partner and a good sense of self, can have a healthy libido despite declining hormones. These factors can potentially change hormonal levels themselves.

Doctors and scientists cannot agree on what percentage of women regularly climax, or how or even *why*. But it's generally accepted that roughly a third of women are unable to have an orgasm through any means, says Cindy

M. Meston, PhD, who was the chair of the World Health Organization's 2005 orgasm committee (yes, there was such a thing). This is one committee I would like to serve on.

One problem is that women have a really hard time lying back and receiving without doing something in return. Oral sex is the ultimate receiving. You start to worry, "It's taking a long time," and then it takes even longer because you're anxious about it.

The reason he's pressuring you to do it is because he wants to give you a gift; this is a way that he's trying to express his love to you. When you're lying there and starting to have those negative thoughts, I encourage you to remember that he's there because he wants to be.

You know what you want, but you're not open to receiving it from *him*. Sometimes that's an issue with the delivery—he can't or won't give you what you want—but sometimes that's about something inside yourself that's closed to him. This isn't about sex. Maybe you are not open to *him*.

A relationship issue may take some soul-searching, some exploring and maybe some therapy to figure out. It certainly can be repaired, but until you feel that connection, you're not going to be open to receiving. Reevaluating your marriage or getting a new boyfriend may allow you to enjoy intense satisfying orgasms.

For many women (and men), masturbation is easier, faster and simply more reliable—like taking the highway versus the scenic country road, says Yvonne K. Fulbright, PhD, sexologist and certified sexuality educator.

You'll be heartened to hear that research has found that women in relationships tend to masturbate more than those who are single. This could be due to many reasons, Fulbright says. "Maybe they're left hanging, or they're exposed to more testosterone through sex, or their partner is unavailable when they're in the mood."

The release of prolactin is 400 times more from orgasms during sex—which tends to make people feel sleepy and satiated—than from those from masturbation, writes Meston in *Why Women Have Sex*, a book she co-authored with psychologist David M. Buss. Still some women prefer masturbation.

However, your super-charged, jelly-rubber vibrator may be causing not only a sexual problem but also a health problem. Some sex toys (seven out of eight in a study by the Netherlands Organization for Applied Scientific Research) contain dangerously high concentrations of phthalates, which are new-car-smelling industrial chemicals that make plastic soft, squishy and easily molded into bumps, ridges and pearls.

Problem is, phthalate exposure—and the genital tract is especially vulnerable—is associated with serious health problems, including hormonal changes and cancers. The jury is out on the chemicals' exact toll on life and libido, but better vibes come from safer materials: medical-grade silicone or rolling a condom over a trusty old rabbit that you suspect has phthalates.

A more natural lubricant is Aloe Cadabra.

There are lots of factors involved in keeping the vagina naturally lubricated, but anything that sabotages your hormone levels or your blood flow throughout the body can make you feel like the Sahara Desert says, Dr. Lauren Streicher.

Elements of natural medicine may help inhibited sexuality. It can be as easy as 1,2,3,4.

Lesson #1: Sexy Foods

Food is love. Food is comfort. Food is sexual enhancement.

Certain foods can enhance your lovemaking. The way a food looks might be visually arousing or psychologically compelling—bonbons and Champagne no doubt conjure up thoughts of seduction and romance.

Consider a Mediterranean diet, which is high in whole grains, fruits, vegetables, fish, and olive oil; a study published in the *International Journal of Impotence Research* found that women who spent two years on this diet experienced a significant boost in their overall sexual function, including arousal. Avoiding your food allergies and/or gluten may give you more energy and highlight sexual experience.

The journey from lifting a fork to increased gratification begins in the brain. "From a psychological standpoint, if you take care of your body by eating well, you'll have a better attitude about sharing it. You'll be more open to sensations and experiences," says Lou Paget, author of several best-selling sex guides, including *The Great Lover Playbook*.[1] "But if a woman eats well, she'll feel better about herself and her sexual attitude can improve immediately," states Paget.

But that's not the only benefit of eating well. "You can absolutely eat your way to better sex. As a rule of thumb, what's good for the heart is good for the genitals," she explains. "If your plumbing—your heart—is clear above the waist, you'll also have better blood flow and more sensation below," says Lynn Edlen-Nezin, Ph.D., a clinical health psychologist and director of behavioral science in New York, and co-author of *Great Food, Great Sex: The Three Food Factors for Sexual Fitness*[2]

There are many foods which (for one reason or another) have a reputation as aphrodisiacs; bananas, avocados, cucumbers, asparagus, oysters, and of course, chocolate and red wine! A diet that includes garlic, ginger, celery, beets, and peanut butter may be just what you need.

According to Julian Whitaker, M.D., founder of Whitaker Wellness Center in Newport Beach, CA, fava beans and soybeans are excellent sources of dopamine, which can enhance sex drive. He recommends increasing intake of these fiber-rich foods to improve libido. Fatty foods can decrease the production of testosterone, the hormone that controls sex drive in both women and men.

Is there scientific evidence? Well, a little. The rest is up to you.

Colorful foods such as spinach, berries, red grapes, peppers and garlic are healthy for you. The healthier you are the more likely you will have sex and enjoy it!

The path to greater sexual satisfaction could begin with eating well balanced nutritious foods, resulting in increased energy and better health. This will get you much closer to your goal of sexual satisfaction and improved intimacy.

Chocolate pumpkin pie (whipped cream optional) is delicious. Beyond the obvious—how can sharing a dessert like pumpkin pie not perk you up?!—there are good reasons to bake your lover a pumpkin pie or order a slice of it instead of another cocktail. In studies conducted by the Smell and Taste Foundation in Chicago, this delectable scent increases blood flow to the penis by forty percent. So why do they just want to watch football on Thanksgiving? I have no idea.

Chocolate just makes everything better, period. Chocolate contains phenylethylamine (a stimulant related to amphetamine) and tryptophan (a building block of serotonin, a brain chemical involved in sexual arousal)—

compounds that are released in the brain when people fall in love. Researchers have noted that the women who like to eat chocolate have a higher libido.

For increased arousal, try watermelon. The compounds present in watermelon may have a "Viagra-like" effect, relaxing blood vessels and increasing blood flow. Proper blood flow allows the tissues to become engorged, aroused and lubricated.

Sexy foods are high in antioxidants, including the popular dark chocolate! In fact, a study of 163 women in *The Journal of Sexual Medicine* found that those who consumed at least one cube of chocolate daily reported significantly greater desire and better overall sexual function than the individuals who abstained - another good reason to eat chocolate.[3] Does chocolate equal better sex? It's always worth trying. Just make sure it is organic, 75 percent chocolate!

Lesson #2: Don't underestimate the power of multivitamins.

A good quality multivitamin that is formulated to exclude wheat, gluten, corn protein, yeast, soy protein, dairy products, nuts, crustacean shellfish, artificial colors, sweeteners, and preservatives, should be your choice. The best quality fish oil should be used that has low mercury risk.

Lesson #3: Consider supplements

Consumerlab.com tested supplements used to enhance male and female sexual performance, and potential benefit was found for only a few of 35 different ingredients. Ginseng, acetyl L-carnitine, DHEA, and Vitamin C. Vitamin C in large doses of 3000 mg was found to enhance women sexually.

Dr. Edlen-Nezin states that nitric oxide (NO) causes blood vessels to expand. "Without an adequate amount of it, guys can't get erections and women can't become engorged and lubricated." Ergo, Dr. Edlen-Nezin suggests that you say yes to L-arginine, an amino acid the body uses to create NO. [4]

Ingesting additional L-arginine has beneficial effects on blood flow, which, in turn, can improve your cardiovascular health, according to a study done in 2001. *The Journal of Clinical Investigation* showed L-arginine significantly improved circulation in young adults with high cholesterol.

Although your coronary arteries are not located in your genitals an assumption can be made that your vessels in that area are dilating as well. L-arginine, an amino acid available in supplement form, may dilate clitoral blood vessels, increasing flow to erogenous zones and helping to improve arousal.

This research is not the definitive word on dietary arginine; Dr. Edlen-Nezin claims that adding it to your diet will improve your sex life. "It can contribute to prolonged arousal." Arginine is found in almonds, walnuts, salmon, cod and halibut.

To get a good mood and keep it, which is essential to wanting to make love in the first place, try rhodiola, a plant-derived supplement. Rhodiola may help block the breakdown of the feel-good hormones dopamine and serotonin. Increasing dopamine can boost female sexual pleasure. Diluting 20-30 drops in a glass of water is the recommended dosage for both men and women.

Zinc is the ultimate sex mineral. Studies show that women with a greater sex drive have higher levels of testosterone. To increase your testosterone, add zinc to your diet. Zinc blocks the enzyme that converts testosterone to estrogen. Pumpkin seeds contain zinc. A quarter-cup serving of pumpkin seeds may do the trick. Zinc increases arousal in women, but to a lesser degree than men.

Ginseng is another long-touted aphrodisiac. Recently, the *Journal of Urology* reported, "the Mean International Index of Erectile Function scores were significantly higher in patients treated with Korean red ginseng than in those who received placebo."[5]

Science and experience have shown sex, smell and taste are related. Alan R. Hirsch, MD, neurological director of the Smell and Taste Treatment and Research Foundation in Chicago, conducted a study that looked at how different smells stimulated sexual arousal.[6] He found that several scents were effective—some more than others. The smell of cheese pizza, for instance, increased blood flow to the penis by five percent, buttered popcorn by nine percent, and lavender and pumpkin pie each by 40 percent.

For women, lavender and pumpkin pie also had a stimulating effect; however, the smell of Good & Plenty® (licorice) combined with the scent of cucumber created the greatest increase in blood flow to the vagina.

There are also herbal products that may enhance libido. If you choose to self- medicate, check with your physician before taking herbs as there are herb-herb interactions and herb-drug interactions. Always make sure you buy the best quality products.

Lesson 4; Your Sexy Brain

It has been said that your brain is your largest sex organ. If your brain is not healthy, your sex life can suffer, too.

Your brain function can affect some basic fundamental aspects of your love life. How you treat that special person in your life, the one important to you in a sexual way, can be a good indicator of your brain's health. A healthy person is a sexual person.

Expressing an unkind remark, shortness of temper, withdrawal of affection, along with other unhappy symptoms, often indicate that your brain chemistry is somehow awry. An unhealthy brain can cause all sorts of mental and physical problems. One of the saddest is the loss of the physical and mental sensations of love and affection that are fundamental to your well-being.

The brain only weighs about three pounds, consists of 60 percent fat and contains 100 billion nerve cells. As each cell has up to 30,000 connections, there are about 1,000 trillion total connections in the brain—more than there are stars in the universe.

No matter what your age or situation, an ever-growing body of research shows that you always have a second chance to shine. The vast majority of women do not want cobwebs in their vaginas.

The brain fitness term suggests that cognitive abilities can be maintained or improved by exercising the brain the same way physical fitness is improved by exercising the body. There is strong evidence that aspects of brain structure remain plastic throughout life, and that high levels of mental activity are associated with reduced risks of confusion, lack of focus, difficulty thinking and age-related dementia.

Eating healthy brain foods like good fats/oils in seeds, nuts, eggs, wild salmon, anchovies, and sardines along with supplements of evening primrose oil and phosphatidylcholine are good for your sex life!

Kissing is good for your health! Researchers at Arizona State University found that frequent kissing reduces stress, improves our bodies' response to and recovery from the stress we do experience, and lowers our levels of bad cholesterol for better heart health. Floyd, K., et al. *Western Journal of Communication, 73*(2), 113–133.

When you're in the middle of a tender kiss, you probably aren't thinking about your waistline. Nevertheless, your kisses are still burning calories. How many depends on the length and passion of each kiss, but a generally accepted rule of thumb is 2 to 6 calories for every minute of kissing. One source, "The Art of Kissing," by William Case, claims that one minute of passionate kissing burns 6.4 calories.

Lesson 5; Exercise for Sex

Do you need motivation to exercise? Did you know that exercise can create female orgasms? Findings from a first-of-its-kind study by Indiana University researchers confirms that exercise (absent of sex or fantasies) can lead to female orgasm.

Exercise-induced orgasms, in particular, seem to have been the gym addict's best-kept secret, until a study late last year by human sexuality researchers at Indiana University revealed that about a quarter of the 530 women they interviewed had climaxed while working on their abdominals, riding a bike or lifting weights.[7]

"While the findings are new, reports of this phenomenon sometimes called "coregasm," because of its association with exercises for core abdominal muscles, have circulated in the media for years," said Debby Herbenick, co-director of the Center for Sexual Health Promotion in Indiana University's School of Health, Physical Education and Recreation. In addition to being a researcher, Herbenick is a widely read advice columnist and book author.

"A healthy, balanced diet sets the table for being sexually satisfied," explains Marrena Lindberg, author of *The Orgasmic Diet: A Revolutionary Plan to Lift Your Libido and Bring You to Orgasm.* "But to get to the next level, you actually have to do a bit more."[8]

So, Lindberg began doing pubococcygeus (PC) exercises, also known as Kegels, to strengthen her weakened vaginal muscles. This is often recommended by OB/GYN physicians to strengthen the pelvic muscles and decrease urinary incontinence.

The surprise result of all these adjustments—Lindberg became spontaneously orgasmic. Spontaneously, as in she was driving her car, listening to the radio, tightening her PC muscles to the beat and then—bam! She climaxed, right there on the highway. My professional advice would be to exercise for vaginal fitness, but not in traffic.

The combination of supplements, dietary changes and vaginal fitness apparently did the trick. Lindberg began an extended period of trial and error, experimenting with dosages and cranking up her PC workout routine until she reached her maximum orgasm potential with her husband. "Now I'm continually orgasmic during sex," she says. "Every three or four thrusts, I have an orgasm—dozens in a row." All of a sudden, supplements, good food, phosphatidylcholine, evening primrose oil and exercise may have "peaked" your interest.

"The most common exercises associated with exercise-induced orgasm were abdominal exercises, climbing poles or ropes, biking/spinning and weight lifting," says Herbenick. "This data is interesting because they suggest that orgasms are not necessarily a sexual event, and that they may also teach us more about the bodily processes underlying women's experiences of orgasm."[9]

We've long known that long-distance bike riding is bad for a man's sex life (heat, pressure, friction = lower sperm count and erectile dysfunction). But women who ride a racing-style bike with handlebars lower than the saddle for more than 10 miles weekly have a serious problem, too finds a study at Texas A&M Health Science Center.

They may lose sensation in their perineum. That sleek, forward-leaning position puts undue pressure on the soft tissues of the perineum and pelvic floor. Riding this way, you may be the hottest, fastest thing on the road but slower to warm up in bed. Better for your sex life is the old fashion 50's style upright.

Here are some key findings:

- About 40 percent of women who had experienced exercise-induced orgasms (EIO) and exercise-induced sexual pleasure (EISP) had done so on more than 10 occasions.
- Most women reporting EIO said they were not fantasizing sexually or thinking about anyone they were attracted to during their experiences.
- Most of the women in the EIO group reported feeling some degree of self-consciousness when exercising in public places, with about 20 percent reporting they could not control their experience.[10]

Yoga and stretching exercises may give you more stamina and positioning options enhancing your sexual experiences.

If you want to enhance your sexual experiences, exercise just might be the answer! On the other hand, too much exercise could wear out most women to the point they could care less about having an orgasm. As an OB/GYN I have heard women complain about exercise, but never because they were having an orgasm in public. They either weren't having the experience or they weren't complaining about it.

Lesson 6: Sex Hormones

What about libido? Once you have had sex with the same person you need a little extra something to go beyond a run-of-the-mill encounter. Do you long for that nonstop passion, instant arousal, running to the bedroom or wherever and ripping your clothes off?

Are you concerned you will start something you cannot finish? Is your will there, but "you" aren't? Dry vaginas are really not appealing either. One of the easiest ways to have moist, healthy tissue in the vagina is to use high dose oral phosphatidylcholine (PC), or you can also insert one capsule of PC into the vagina to heal and soften the tissues.

When giving patients intravenous phosphatidylcholine it was soon apparent that there was an interesting 'side effect.' Libido is so sharply increased that many patients (both men and women) comment on the effect.

There are many foods and herbs that mitigate menopausal symptoms and relieve dry vaginas. The volume of these options is beyond the scope of this book. However, a report out of Cleveland, Ohio is that oat straw is very effective. Oat straw promotes vaginal lubrication. Use one teaspoon of the herb infused in one cup of water for 10 minutes. Drink three times a day as a tonic.

A lack of lubrication can turn into a waning sex drive because natural lubrication is a primary signal of arousal. You want to be friction-free. Aloe Cadabra is an all natural lubricant that contains certified organic ingredients. It is free of harmful petroleum products and parabens. Be wet and healthy.

In a study at Southwestern University in Georgetown, Texas, scientists increased libido in female test subjects by giving them caffeine. Granted, the test subjects were rats.[11]

The sex hormones estrogen, progesterone, and testosterone are keys to increased libido and orgasms. The other "dancing hormones" such as thyroid and cortisol along with balanced neurotransmitters are the foundation for good health and good sex!

In the months leading up to menopause, estrogen levels drop, which can cause vaginal dryness—often a painful turnoff. But there's a simple solution: Talk to your gynecologist about using a topical bio-identical estrogen cream to banish dryness quickly and make sex fun again.

Forty percent of women will experience a decline in libido. Well before women hit menopause, their bodies begin to make changes that affect hormone levels. The ovaries, which are the source of 50% of our testosterone, become less active, decreasing the production of the sex hormone that is key to our libido.

Testosterone is a female hormone produced by the ovaries and adrenal glands. As estrogen decreases, so does testosterone. Women may need testosterone replacement with the estrogen and progesterone in the menopause. It's this decline in testosterone that's really responsible for a reduced sex drive and orgasms.

Speaking of orgasms, have you ever wondered how long an intense orgasm lasts? According to sex researchers Masters and Johnson it involves 8 to 12 vaginal contractions, each lasting 4.0 to 9.6 seconds. That adds up to over two minutes of continuous mind-bending bliss.

Are you too cold to climax? That's cold not old. Men aren't the only ones whose extremities need warming up. Women's do, too—down there, *way* down there. In an orgasm study at the University of Groningen, half the couples were unable to make it to climax.

According to the research, it was cold feet! Once socks were offered, the success rate shot up to 80 percent. Comfort is key—and the area of the brain associated with genital sensation is right next-door to the one associated with feeling in the feet, writes Daniel Amen, MD, in his book *Unleash the Power of the Female Brain*.

Oxytocin is an important hormone to consider. It decreases anxiety, increases happiness and love. It has also been shown to increase the intensity of organisms! All good things.

A decline in the level of hormones is neither irreparable nor permanent.

Low testosterone is one reason for erectile dysfunction (and low libido in women). Chronic illness is another; asthma, diabetes, lack of exercise, inflammation, obesity, fatigue, depression and, prostate surgery.

You remember the spontaneous erections, firm intense desire and lasting stamina. For your mind and body to respond to sex like a well-oiled, orgasm-primed machine you need to be healthy and energetic.

Evening Primrose oil stimulates prostaglandin E1 which is science behind stimulating erections in males and orgasms in both men and women.

Stress in your life can also lead to low libido. You may have already instinctively felt this with high cortisol, epinephrine, and nor-epinephrine.

Exercising to build muscle mass usually will increase testosterone levels, too, which may be another reason why exercise increases sex drive. According to *Discovery Health*, "Moderate regular exercise will help improve blood flow to the sexual organs. In addition, exercise helps you feel good about yourself. Anything that improves self-esteem will improve libido."[12]

The right hormonal balance, nutrition and exercise can put that bounce back in your step again!

If you have a healthy mind, body and spirit, but still find yourself with decreased sexual desires and arousal, you may have declining or a deficiency in estrogen, progesterone and/or testosterone. This deficiency is most common in menopause or if the woman has experienced a surgical menopause. Consult with your physician about the risks and benefits of using bio-identical hormone replacement therapy.

Once you have the information, consider your family's health history as well as your own. Add to this information your own personal preference and make a knowledgeable decision regarding hormonal replacement therapy. If the answer is yes, the next step is to decide if you want to use a commercially available product or bio-identical hormones?

Bio-identical hormones are structurally identical to the hormones produced by the human body and are intended to replace these hormones when levels decline as a consequence of aging, disease or surgery. Customization through a compounding pharmacy can maximize the therapeutic effects while minimizing the potential for adverse effects.

Studies show that 65% of women with low levels of testosterone who take supplemental testosterone increase their libido, sexual response, energy and have a better sense of overall well-being.

What about the men?

Penis is an anatomical term…and, of course, much more. The penis is a barometer of your health status.

But male sexual dysfunction is *not* a natural part of aging. When there is trouble "down there" there may be trouble elsewhere. What are the causes of a slow penis? It may mean your blood vessels are clogged from atherosclerosis. It may also mean you have nerve damage from diabetes.

Problems with erections may stem from medications, chronic illnesses, hormonal imbalance, mood disorders, poor blood flow to the penis, drinking too much alcohol, or being too tired.

If you have difficulty achieving or maintaining an erection, you may want to take a look inside your medicine cabinet. Medications account for 25 percent of ED.

Medications can create ED but the medications are a reflection that you are not in good health, and as a result your penis is affected.

Additional steps to enhancing your libido.

- Communication. Simply setting aside time to talk with your partner is a good start. Picking the right time and right place for this discussion is key to success.

- Mood. Women often take responsibility for getting into the mood. Giving yourself a day without decisions, demands or deadlines is a great way to create the mood.
- Intimacy. Take time for the personal connection
- Sensuality. Consider the sight of the bedroom and your personal preferences for smell, touch, taste and sound.
- Passion. Remember, the brain is the biggest sex organ in the body. Talk to your partner, be vulnerable, take risks and laugh together.

Lesson 7; Sex improves health and longevity.

Here is why science suggests you should get frisky tonight.

"The key," says Carl J. Charnetski, PhD, "lies in the production of natural opioid peptides—happy little brain chemicals that are released during sex and in turn boost production of IGA, a protein from the immune system." Carl J. Charnetski, PhD, is the Professor of Psychology at Wilkes University and author of the book, *Feeling Good is Good for You; How Pleasure can Boost Your Immune System*. This is a natural approach to avoiding colds and the flu.[13] This could also prove to be a good pick up line. "I would like to help you avoid getting a cold or the flu."

The surge of oxytocin that occurs during orgasm triggers a release of feel-good endorphins that act as powerful pain relievers. The orgasm cure can also work on arthritis, backaches and muscle pain.

Any medical expert—nutritionist, sex researcher, internist, heart surgeon— will tell you that the best things to eat for a healthy love life are also the best things for a healthy heart. As Dr. Oz has repeatedly stressed, when your arteries are clogged and your circulation is impaired, blood can't flow to where it needs to go, and in this case, it *needs* to get to your genitals.

According to Dr. Oz we already know that sex can be a decent cardio workout (one 30-minute session can burn 70 calories); now research indicates it may protect your heart in other ways.

A study in the *Journal of Sex & Marital Therapy* found that people who had sex an average of 12 times per month had greater heart rate variability (HRV)—a measure of how well the heart responds to subtle changes throughout the day (like standing versus sitting). Higher HRV is a good thing; it may lower your risk of developing heart disease, the leading cause of death for women.

For women, quality trumps quantity when it comes to the lifesaving effects of sex. Simply having positive memories about your sexual past may add roughly four years to your life, according to research at the Duke Center for the Study of Aging and Human Development. Researchers found that these fond memories may encourage you to continue leading a happier, healthier life.

Being in a healthy, fulfilling sexual relationship can do wonders for your overall wellness. Yet about 7 percent of married people and 17.7 percent of partnered people in their 30s and 40s say they haven't had sex in the past year, according to the 2010 National Survey of Sexual Health and Behavior.

Whether you find that comforting or alarming, Fulbright reminds you of the fringe benefits of getting busy: Sex improves the muscle tone of the pelvic floor, lubricates the vaginal tissues, can help prevent yeast infections, releases stress, and eases migraines, chronic back pain and PMS-related cramps. Sex also has the potential for lowering your risk of developing heart disease, boosting your immune system, and making you look younger.

Roughly 53 percent of Americans say they're too worn out at the end of the day to fool around, according to a poll by Consumer Reports. To power up your sex life, consider powering down your electronic gadgets.

New research indicates that the backlight from the screens of electronics may be the reason you're not getting a good night's rest (the light tricks the brain by simulating daylight, making you less likely to fall asleep). A study by the Lighting Research Center at Rensselaer Polytechnic Institute found that two hours of watching TV before bed suppressed melatonin—the hormone responsible for regulating your sleep schedule—by about 23 percent.

Did you know that having more sex can increase your life expectancy? It's true! Sex releases several hormones such as estrogen and oxytocin throughout the body, increasing intimacy and bonding. Staying sexually active has physical, stress-relieving, social and mental benefits.

Frequent orgasms (about 100 per year) can increase life expectancy by three to eight years; however, keep in mind that the science on this is somewhat spotty. Studies show that men with a high frequency of orgasms have a 50 percent reduction in mortality risk. Sexual activity seems to have a protective affect on men's health.[14] It also helps fight against loneliness and depression.

In an Arizona State University study on 58 middle-aged women, physical affection or sexual behavior with a partner significantly predicted lower negative mood and stress and higher positive mood the following day. Simply put, researchers found that sex and physical intimacy led women to feel less stressed and be in a better mood the next day. (These results weren't found when women had orgasms without a partner.)[15]

Not only do women live longer and feel better but they look better! Here's a prescription: Have sex at least three times a week. In a study at Scotland's Royal Edinburgh Hospital, people in their 40s who reported having an average of 50 percent more sex than the typical person were judged by a panel of strangers to be about seven to 13 years younger than their actual age.

Researchers believe the youthful glow comes in part from the release of the DHEA hormone during sex. DHEA, which is produced by your adrenal glands, has antiaging properties that can increase the production of collagen and may reduce wrinkles.

Some of my patients would not agree with this report. This study reminds me of one of them. In the waiting room the subject of her husband came up. She said to my receptionist and me, "Well, if things don't work out, I will be so happy with my cat and my vibrator."

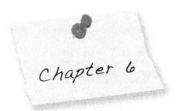

Chapter 6

MOODS: FINDING
THE ROOT CAUSE

The mind really matters.

We've all heard the saying, "When Mom's not happy, no one is happy." A parent's struggle with emotional imbalance affects not only the parent but the entire family. Depression, anxiety and mood swings are not something you can just "snap out of." Science proves these disorders can be caused by an imbalance of brain chemicals, along with other mitigating factors. Treatment usually includes rounds of psychotherapy or treatment with an array of pharmaceutical drugs. There are better solutions than drugs.

Physicians have been taught to "name or blame" a disease, then find a matching pharmaceutical drug in an attempt to relieve the symptoms. Today, however, we've learned that there is no such thing as a single disease, but rather underlying causes of an illness or imbalances that create disease. This explains why people are often diagnosed with multiple mood disorders or symptoms and they get sicker and sicker.

People's brains are broken. They know it. They feel it. They live it. If they have a physical disease, it may be obvious. They may not be able to hide it. On the other hand, many suffer in silence with mood disorders, "psychiatric disease," and memory loss. The symptoms of lack of motivation, fatigue, lack of focus, and brain fog may be viewed as character flaws. Instead they are often neurotransmitter or hormonal imbalances that can be corrected.

With the onslaught of so much stress and so many chemical and other environmental challenges, it is no wonder that our bodies are challenged and our brains are broken.

Anxiety and depression may seem like polar opposites, but in truth, they can be very similar and are often linked.

Today, clinical depression is the leading cause of disability with 20 million Americans suffering and 30 million pharmaceutical drugs prescribed, according to the *Archives of General Psychiatry*.[1]

Major depressive disorder (MDD) is a debilitating illness affecting about 12% of men and 25% of women. It lasts more than 2 years in 30 percent of patients.

Sadly, depression is only one of many symptoms observed when there are neurotransmitter imbalances.

At a recent national medical conference, Dr. Robert J. Hedaya, Founder of the National Center for Whole Psychiatry and Clinical Professor of Psychiatry at Georgetown University, reviewed the evolution of the model of mood disorders:

- Middle Ages: Demons within—exorcism is the treatment of choice.
- 1917: Freud explains that the so-called 'demons within' are really our mothers.
- 1988: Eli Lilly releases our mothers from 80 years of victimization, explaining that depression is really a Prozac deficiency.

Dr. Hedaya's humor draws attention to the current model of therapy for mood disorders. The problem is that the model only works partially sometimes, and often causes additional problems. Treating mood disorders is based on sequential augmentation strategies.

Psychological stress and physiological changes can cause neurotransmitter deficiencies or imbalances; likewise, the neurotransmitter deficiency or imbalance can cause psychological stress and physiological changes. Fortunately, neurotransmitters can be measured by specialized laboratory testing.

Psychiatrists are the only medical specialists that do not test the organ they treat—the brain! Internists and family doctors also, rarely if ever, test neurotransmitters before pulling out the prescription pad. Doctors often prescribe Zoloft®, Lexapro®, Paxil®, Wellbutrin®, Celexa®, Prozac® and other mood-alerting drugs. If they don't work, they may increase the dose. If that doesn't work they may change to another drug, and if that doesn't work they may add another drug to the first, or maybe they will add a third or a fourth and soon the patients may show signs of being bipolar.

Conventional medical protocol is to order a lab before prescribing pharmaceutical drugs. Think of it this way—it is a common practice to measure thyroid levels before prescribing medication. The same is true for cholesterol and most other conditions. Therefore, before treating an individual with neurotransmitter imbalances, it makes sense to test the level of the neurotransmitters. Specialty tests can identify specific levels so the health care practitioner can recommend the best therapeutic support and the right supplements to balance the neurotransmitters.

To observe American society today, one might believe there is a massive epidemic of Prozac dependence. Doctors are doling out the anti-depressants like candy even though anxiety and depression may be caused by nutrient or bio-chemical deficiencies.

Neurotransmitters are chemicals used to replay, amplify and modulate electrical signals between the nerve cells and other cells. The brain makes over 100 of these chemical messengers that are produced and stored in the brain and released into action when the brain cells are electrically activated. They are responsible for every thought, mood, pain and pleasure sensation we feel. They control our energy level, our appetite and the foods we crave. Neurotransmitters even regulate how well we sleep as well as our sex drive.

Irregularities in this system result in hormonal imbalances and multiple symptoms, which can cause dramatic effects on our daily life.

Millions of Americans are experiencing depression and unhappiness, yet commonly they are simply prescribed the band-aid of a pharmaceutical drug. It is important to find the underlying causes of these issues while using natural therapies to support biochemical balance.

The most commonly prescribed medications are selective serotonin re-uptake inhibitors (SSRIs). These include Prozac®, Paxil®, Zoloft®, Effexor®, Serafem®, Serzone®, Celexa® and Lexapro®. Research has shown their effectiveness to be approximately 30 percent, which was often equal to a placebo. According to Dr. Hedaya, by the researchers a mood-altering drug is considered effective if it reduces symptoms of depression by 50 percent.

To get FDA approval for a drug, two clinical trial presentations are required to show that the drug is effective. The pharmaceutical company needed to conduct seven clinical trials to find two that showed the effectiveness of Paxil. Those two clinical trials were presented to the FDA and received approval to go to the market.

These drugs are thought to work by regulating some neurotransmitters, but unfortunately, they impair critical pathways resulting in well-known side effects. These are "universal" drugs prescribed for persons without testing to determine the individual's levels of serotonin, dopamine, GABA, nor-epinephrine (NE), epinephrine (E), glutamate and/or cortisol.

Serotonin Selective Reuptake Inhibitors (SSRIs), a common class of drugs that support regulation of serotonin by altering the way the brain functions, help 30 to 50 percent of the time, but also have side effects 86 percent of the time. Known adverse effects include, but are not limited to the following:

- Increased suicide risk (acutely) in children and adolescents
- Weight gain
- Sexual dysfunction
- Emotional detachment
- Twice the annual rate of bone loss (vs. tricyclic antidepressants)
- Withdrawal
- Induction of mania, agitation, aggression, paranoia
- Suicide rates increase in children under the age of 18

Dr. Watkins Monograph stated in *Managing Depression and Anxiety-Providing Options and Adjuncts to Pharmaceutical Treatments,* "In a study looking at all the studies that were brought to the FDA regarding 4 new generation anti-depressants published in 2008, only those patients at the upper end of the very severely depressed category seemed to receive any benefit from their drug treatment compared to placebo. We also know from the literature that remission rates (that is, those who get better) run in the 20–30 percent range for most studies—even when "depression care specialists" are involved in the treatment programs—while most patients have either no or little improvement with anti-depressant treatment."[2,3]

Dr. Erick Turner, a professor of psychiatry at Oregon Health and Science University shook up the medical community and the pharmaceutical industry in January 2008 by his paper, *Selective Publication of Antidepressant Trials and Its Influence on Apparent Efficacy* in the *New England Journal of Medicine.* This paper showed that the antidepressants are not as effective as the drug companies would like us to think. He looked at 74 clinical trials. Of those, 51 percent found that a drug had performed better than a placebo (a sugar pill), while 49 percent were negative or had mixed results.

Most of the negative results were never published. The trials showing positive results were published. The physicians, patients, public, and the media had misinformation. The pharmaceutical drug companies had overstated the effectiveness of their pills for two decades. If a study showed the placebo was more effective than the drug, the trial was never published. The drugs were made to appear more beneficial than they really were.

This can lead to doctors making 'inappropriate prescribing decisions' which is not the right care. In spite of this information available since 2008, "The CDC's National Center for Health Statistics reports that the rate of antidepressant use in the U.S. has increased nearly 400 percent since 1988."[4]

The good news is that advances in science have made it possible for individuals to not only measure their neurotransmitters, but to correct deficiencies and imbalances. Happiness and optimal health have their own biochemistry, which can be powerfully balanced and enhanced naturally. Many alternative methods aimed at raising neurotransmitter levels have been widely used with reported significant success.

These methods include acupuncture, hypnosis, massage, reflexology, meditation, yoga, and natural supplements. Research has also shown that walking briskly each day is as effective as Prozac for depression. In fact, neurotransmitter measurements conducted on meditating Tibetan monks showed increased levels of serotonin—the "serenity" messenger.[5]

With the scientific data now supporting the benefits of these ancient treatments, more western medical disciplines are becoming convinced and subsequently integrating them into treatment protocols.

Since a neurotransmitter imbalance may create or exacerbate mood disorders, testing the neurotransmitters before treatment provides information for the physician and the patient to customize treatment. "Treating the average" is overrated. We wouldn't give someone insulin unless we knew their current blood sugar levels. We wouldn't give thyroid medication unless we knew what the existing thyroid levels were. Why would we treat mood disorders without measuring neurotransmitters in advance?

Low Levels of Neurotransmitters

Neurotransmitters and hormones commonly measured are serotonin, epinephrine, GABA, dopamine, nor-epinephrine, glutamate, cortisol, DHEA and thyroid. A deficiency of any particular neurotransmitter not only affects neuronal function, but also endocrine function anywhere in the body.

Our endocrine system is considered primary and critical to all metabolic function. Glands such as the thyroid, the adrenals, the ovaries and the testes all take direction from the brain. There are many conditions that negatively impact hormone levels, and when one hormone is imbalanced, there is a tendency for many other hormones to follow suit. Correction of imbalanced hormones is important but not always sufficient. The correction of imbalanced neurotransmitters, on the other hand, is imperative if clinical progress is to be made. Determining which neurotransmitters are low and which are high should precede clinical intervention.

Is your doctor testing?

Combining poor diet with a stressful life-style is a recipe for serotonin depletion. The types of food we crave (starches, chocolate or sweets) and the time of day we crave them (late afternoon or evening) may characterize specific neurotransmitter deficiencies. In fact, serotonin depletion is one of the most common neurotransmitter imbalances in our culture.

Low Serotonin
Anxiety
Panic attacks
Depression
Insomnia
PMS
Hot flashes
Headaches
Pain
Low libido
Constipation
Carbohydrate cravings
Fatigue

Low Epinephrine
Lack of focus
Poor blood sugar control
Difficulty losing weight

Low GABA
Anxiety
Hyperactivity
Excess worrying
Insomnia

Dopamine is the euphoric NT. It is how we see the world. It gives meaning to life. Low dopamine is a factor in drug addictions and relapse.

Low Dopamine

Increased risk of addictions

Cravings

Lack of focus

Low motivation

Low libido

Lacking joy and meaning to life

Low Nor-epinephrine

Lack of focus

Decreased energy

Depression with apathy

Lack of energy

Poor methylation

Low Glutamate

Fatigue

Low brain function

High Levels of Neurotransmitters

High levels of neurotransmitters (NT) have their own symptoms—these elevations are increased when calming inhibitory NT like serotonin and GABA are low. It is a balancing act.

High Epinephrine

Stress

Anxiety

Insomnia

Lack of focus

Lack of energy

Blood sugar elevation
Insulin resistance

High Nor-epinephrine
Stress
Anxiety
Hyperactivity
ADD and ADHD
Anger
Pain
Increased blood pressure
Migraines
Hot flashes

High Glutamate
Stress
Anxiety
Depressed mood
Neurotoxicity
Seizures

What causes neurotransmitter deficiencies?

Weight-Loss Dieting

Dieting is the most common cause of self-induced neurotransmitter deficiencies.[6] Protein-deficient diets may not supply adequate tryptophan, which is necessary for serotonin production. Carbohydrates assist in the delivery of tryptophan to the brain for serotonin production. High protein/ low carbohydrate diets are a two-fold problem—there is not enough insulin and too much amino acid competition, which restricts the basic building blocks needed to produce enough neurotransmitters.[7]

Studies from major universities, including Harvard, MIT and Oxford, have documented that women on diets significantly deplete their serotonin within three weeks of dieting![8] This induced serotonin deficiency may eventually lead to increased cravings, moodiness and poor motivation, which all contribute to rebound weight gain—the common yet unfortunate consequence of dieting. Low dopamine can sabotage weight control.

Diets may also be deficient in B-vitamins and other necessary nutrients. Folinic acid, B6, and magnesium are all required in the process of serotonin production. Therefore, it is so important to see a health care professional for your weight-loss program where you have the opportunity for neurotransmitter support that can help ensure successful weight loss with a healthy program specifically designed for you.

Certain Medications

Long term use of diet pills, stimulants, pain pills, narcotics and recreational drugs can deplete neurotransmitter stores. Diet pills (like phen-fen, phenteramine) use up large amounts of dopamine and serotonin, which can result in "rebound" appetite control problems, low energy, unstable moods and a sluggish metabolism.[7]

Prolonged Emotional or Physical Stress

The human body is designed to handle sudden, acute or short bouts of stress. Prolonged chronic stress takes its toll on the "fight or flight" stress hormones and neurotransmitters. Eventually, these hormones and neurotransmitters become depleted and coping with stress becomes more difficult.

Aging

Sixty percent of all adults over the age of 40 have some degree of neurotransmitter deficiencies. Aging brain cells make smaller amounts of neurotransmitters. Also, as we get older, the body does not respond as well to them. Balancing the NT helps to maintain a more youthful brain and body.

Abnormal Sleep

Stressors of all sorts can become chronic and cause adrenal fatigue. Many neurotransmitters are responsible for proper sleep, especially serotonin. It is produced during REM sleep around 2am to 3am when serotonin converts to melatonin, the sleep hormone. When serotonin levels are low, melatonin levels will also be low. The result is disrupted sleep. Sleepless nights also contribute to other NT imbalances which in turn compounds the lack of a good night's sleep.

Toxicity

Mercury, lead, aluminum, cadmium and arsenic are major neurotoxins. Chemical pesticides, fertilizers, certain cleaning agents, industrial solvents and recreational drugs cause damage to the brain cells and decrease neurotransmitter production.[8]

Inflammation

Any condition ending in "itis", such as sinusitis, gastritis or arthritis is an inflammatory condition. Inflammation interferes with the conversion of tryptophan to 5-HTP which is used in the body's production of serotonin.[9] 5-HTP is a blood chemical that works in the brain by increasing the production of serotonin.

Serotonin is made from 5-HTP. Numerous double-blind studies have shown 5-HTP to be as effective as prescription antidepressants but more tolerable. Another placebo-controlled study has shown tyrosine to also be as effective as antidepressants supporting dopamine and NE without side effects.[10] It is important to note that these effective supplements should not be used when taking a SSRI. In addition, if 5-HTP is given without tyrosine, it often stops working after a few months. Taking tyrosine along with the 5-HTP will result in long-lasting improvement.

Have you tried 5-HTP and it didn't work? When buying 5-HTP or other supplements over the counter or on the internet it has been shown that 40–50 percent of the time they may contain contaminants and 40–50 percent of the time they may not contain what the label indicates. Quality 5-HTP in targeted nutrient therapies has been shown to be effective. It is important to also have sufficient vitamin B6 as it is needed to convert 5-HPT to serotonin.

Serotonin is the calming happy hormone. We all need normal levels to be happy, healthy, energetic and productive.

Inflammation is the underlying cause of most chronic diseases.[10] Too much or too little inflammation creates disease. Inflammation of the brain is a central theme for almost all psychiatric and neurologic conditions. Gluten, food allergens, infections, toxins, sugar and mold create inflammation. When you cool your inflammation, you can heal your brain.

Hormonal Imbalance

If hormones are deficient or are off-balance, neurotransmitters do not function well. Premenstrual Syndrome (PMS) is a classic example of how low estrogen levels can shift each month. Estrogen and serotonin support each other, so when the estrogen level is low, the signs and symptoms of low serotonin are apparent. Mood, appetite and sleep can be severely disrupted one to two weeks before the menstrual cycle.

Neurotransmitter imbalances occur during menopause when dramatic changes in mood, energy, sleep, weight and sexual desire occur. Thyroid and cortisol also impact the neurotransmitter balance. Our hormones, including insulin, thyroid, sex hormones, stress hormones, and neurotransmitters are a symphony of molecules. They work in harmony for you to be healthy. Think of them as dancing partners!

Genetic Predisposition

Some people are born with a limited ability to make adequate amounts of neurotransmitters. These individuals exhibit deficiency symptoms as children or young adults and often have relatives who suffer from significant mental illnesses. As they age, affected individuals experience even more profound symptoms and debilitation.

Once the imbalances are identified through laboratory testing of specific neurotransmitters, individuals can correct the imbalances through psychological support and treatments. There are many ways to correct these imbalances including, but are not limited to, lifestyle changes, hormone balancing, nutrition, supplements, and pharmaceuticals if indicated. The key is to test the NT through specialized lab testing and then use specific targeted amino acids and nutrients to balance the NTs. It is natural, effective and without side effects.

Clearly, neurotransmitter imbalance has multiple causes and dramatic effects on our daily life. One of the foundations for a healthy and harmonious family is balanced neurotransmitters.

Is your doctor testing neurotransmitters so you can be treated as an individual?

Nutrition for the brain

About two-thirds of our brain is made of fat. Consequently, nerve and brain function are dependent on lipids. Essential fatty acids are crucial for normal brain function which include both omega 3 fatty acids as alpha-linoleic acid (flaxseed, hempseed oil) and EPA/DHA (fish oil, wild salmon, sardines, anchovies) and omega 6 linoleic acid (organic sunflower, safflower, hempseed), gamma linolenic acid (evening primrose oil from Canada), and arachidonic acid (egg yolk, organic butter and meat fat).

Dietary corrections are also important for restoring healthy brain function, but may not be enough to correct a significant neurotransmitter deficiency since foods can vary in their nutrient content and intestinal absorption can be unpredictable. Most neurotransmitters are made from protein, i.e., amino acids. A safe and effective way to raise neurotransmitter levels is to give your body the building blocks it needs to make them.

It goes without saying that nutritional support is also essential. Neurotransmitter health must be maintained with a balanced diet that includes adequate amounts of protein, carbohydrates and good fats. Eating adequate amounts of protein is critical and the average person requires 40 to 70 grams of protein daily.[11]

No food group should be eliminated since they are all critical for proper neurotransmitter production and function. Dietary toxins such as excess caffeine, nicotine, alcohol and sugar create imbalances and should be avoided.

Furthermore, approximately one third of patients with depression have been found to be deficient in folinic acid, which can cause depression as can

B12 deficiency.[12] Depression is also a common symptom of deficiency in the B-vitamins riboflavin and niacin, which are critical for energy production. Vitamin B6 levels, critical in the production of serotonin, dopamine and NE, are generally quite low in depressed patients, and this is especially problematic for women taking birth control pills or estrogen—both of which can deplete vitamin B6 levels.

Magnesium deficiency is the single most relevant nutritional deficiency in the United States today.[13,14] The average Chinese diet contains approximately 650 mg of magnesium a day, compared to the average American diet substantially loaded with processed food and containing roughly 250 mg. This contributes to pain, fatigue and increased risk of heart attacks, depression and numerous other problems, as magnesium is critical for the 300 different reactions in the body. Low levels of vitamin D have also been shown to lead to depression.[15]

A recent article in the International Journal of Neuropsychiatric Medicine (2009) by Andrew Farah, MD reviews the research for the effectiveness for the use of L-methylfolate as approach to depression. The key here is to use the methylated form of folic acid as the body is better able to use it supporting serotonin, norepinephrine, and dopamine.

Serotonin originates from the amino acid tryptophan, which is the least common amino acid in food. It is also the most difficult to absorb into the brain. Eating tryptophan-rich foods like fish, turkey, dairy products, eggs, nuts, seeds and wheat germ will not substantially increase serotonin levels because these foods contain other amino acids that compete with tryptophan for absorption and win!

Surprisingly, eating carbohydrates raises serotonin levels, but eating protein decreases serotonin. Carbohydrates cause an insulin response that favors tryptophan absorption over the other amino acids. This explains why many people who need serotonin (like those who are overly-stressed or depressed) start to "self-medicate" by eating more sweets. As the tryptophan rises, so will serotonin production. Serotonin is the main neurotransmitter for mood and appetite regulation and depends on carbohydrates for its production. Seventy percent of people with low serotonin also have insomnia and 71 percent have pain.[16]

Furthermore, studies from Harvard, MIT and Oxford Universities demonstrate that women on high protein/very low carbohydrate diets lower their serotonin levels making them more prone to weight gain relapse, depression, excessive craving, binging, bulimia, severe PMS and seasonal affective disorder.

Solutions for Your Brain

How do you find out what is best for you in maintaining optimum health and balancing the complex interdependent neurotransmitters and hormones?

- First, determine your neurotransmitter/hormonal levels through specialty lab tests.
- Second, use specific targeted nutrient therapies to balance your neurotransmitters.

Treatment may include various natural supplements. Imbalances can be corrected with amino acids, IV therapies for detoxification and other nutrients. Balanced essential fatty acids, phosphatidylcholine, a quality multivitamin, Vitamin D and the B vitamins (the anti-stress vitamins) may also be recommended. Magnesium, manganese, chromium, zinc, calcium, copper, iron and potassium are minerals that support brain function, while pharmaceutical drugs simply mask the problems.

Nutritional support, exercise or other healing practices have been shown to be beneficial to balancing neurotransmitters and hormones. You *can* feel so much better!

Our bodies function using the air we breathe, the water we drink and the food we eat. Our brains are broken because of poor diet, environmental allergens and toxins, auto-immune diseases, infections and stress. These factors not only change our bio-chemistry but change the function of our genes as well.

Nothing damages the brain more than stress. Stress can shrink the brain. Stress increases inflammation just like sugar. Gradually the brain fog settles in.

For great information on inflammation, read Dr. Mark Hyman's *Blood Sugar Solution*.

The Brain Can Heal

The brain can be revitalized with targeted nutritional support. We should not accept the pain and suffering of mental illness, stress, mood changes and psychiatric challenges as something to endure or be embarrassed about in ourselves or our loved ones. These disorders are the result of imbalanced neurochemistry and may be addressed from a cellular perspective to achieve normal mental function.

Point #1: Brain Food

As the brain is 60 percent lipid it is paramount to focus on balanced, essential fatty acids to support mental function. High quality protein is also crucial to support the brain as it supplies amino acids for neurotransmitters, enzymes and molecular structures. What about pasta, bread and sugar? They just plain taste good—yet, carbs do not support brain health, and they often create the problem by stimulating enzymes that provoke the breakdown of phospholipids in the cell membranes.

It is key to also avoid any foods you are allergic to and avoid gluten if you have gluten sensitivity.

Many people with emotional challenges have gross imbalances in their cellular fatty acid content, most commonly a severe suppression of total lipid content. Red cell lipid testing is available to identify the exact balance that you need, or you can use a balance of essential fatty acids in your diet and through supplementation to regain stability. I use an excellent lab at Johns Hopkins for a comprehensive essential fatty acid report.

The most powerful tool you have to change your brain and your health is what you eat.

A diet high in essential fatty acid with supportive supplementation as phosphatidylcholine, the short chain fatty acid butyrate, evening primrose oil, high EPA fish oil, hempseed oil or 4:1 omega 6 (linoleic acid to omega 3 alpha linolenic acid) and arachidonic acid (egg yolk, organic butter) directly affects and optimizes cellular and brain function to support the healing process.

Point # 2: Balance Hormones and Neurotransmitters

Our hormones are stabilized by a proper balance of essential fatty acids. Insulin is pivotal to healthy mental responses and is controlled with a diet high in nutrient dense foods, essential fatty acids and protein with limited carbohydrate intake. All the hormones, including the thyroid, sex hormones and stress hormones work in unison with neurotransmitters and prostaglandins (essential fatty acids) which act as a symphony of molecules.

"We have found that if a drug can be found to do the job of medical healing, a nutrient can be found to do the same job. We now know that if we give the amino acids, the body will synthesize neurotransmitters, thereby achieving the same effect as drugs. The challenge of the future is to replace drugs with these natural healers", stated Dr. Carl Pfeiffer, a pioneer amino-acid researcher.

Neurotransmitters are supplied from the high quality protein that we consume but for some, impaired digestion of protein, stress, and vitamin/mineral depletion limit their availability. Testing urinary neurotransmitters can be very helpful and guide your physician to suggest supportive amino acid supplementation specific to your needs.

Point # 3: Blunt Inflammation

Inflammation may be a complicating factor that can be boldly addressed by removing all sugar and if possible all grains (wheat, oat, rice, rye, corn) from the diet. Inflammation can lead to edema and edema may lead to a swollen brain. Reducing carbohydrates while increasing balanced lipids and protein controls insulin and membrane breakdown. Infections and toxins such as mold can also create inflammation. The use of phosphatidylcholine and the short chain fatty acid butyrate clears inflammation and are primary nutrients towards healing your brain.

Point # 4: Support Absorption of Nutrients

The gastrointestinal (GI) tract is called our "second brain" as described by Columbia University physician, Michael Gershon in his book, *The Second Brain*.[17] The GI tract has as many neurons (brain cells) as the main frame brain and has more neurons than the spinal column. Neurotransmitters, including 95 percent of serotonin, are produced in the GI tract. Clearly, digesting, absorbing and assimilating all the food and nutrients we eat are critical for our brains and overall health.[19] The GI tract also has the ability to detoxify and contains 70 percent of our immune system. Your GI tract must be healthy for your whole body to be healthy.

Caring for our second brain which functions to digest, absorb and assimilate all the food and nutrients we consume is crucial for our brain as it is for our overall health. Support using betaine or HCl, digestive enzymes, and probiotic supplements are necessary for some individuals to maximize GI function.

Keeping the bowels open is also an important part of healing so that wastes and toxins can be eliminated properly.

Point # 5: Clear Toxins
Neurotoxicity is a major aspect of why our brains do not perform optimally. Brain fog, memory difficulties, mental fatigue, anxiety, depression, rage, mood swings, and even psychosis can result from toxic assault. In some cases it is necessary to use intravenous phosphatidylcholine, folinic acid, and glutathione to expedite the removal of toxins.

Point # 6: Supporting Mitochondrial /Energy Cellular Metabolism
We often think of fatigue as something we experience in the physical body, however the brain also requires liberal amounts of energy; approximately 20 percent of the body's total energy is required for mental function. Feeding the mitochondria with phosphatidylcholine and linoleic acid (organic sunflower or safflower oil) nourishes the inner membrane of mitochondria. Nutrients such as manganese and CoQ10 are also supportive to mitochondrial, energy production.

Point # 7: Joy and Laughter
Keep your sense of humor and laugh a lot! A life of meaning and purpose, a life in balance with connection, community, love, support and a sense of empowerment are essential for health. The overwhelming stresses, such as

social isolation, over-work and disempowerment, create enormous strain on our nervous systems, leading to burnout and breakdown.

The brain produces more than 100 neurotransmitters, which control every thought, mood, pain and pleasure sensation we feel, as well as our energy level, motivation, appetite and cravings. Neurotransmitters even regulate how well we sleep, our sex drive and our ability to focus and concentrate. When out of balance, mood disorders and addictions can result.

Find the underlying cause of your neurotransmitter imbalance or mood disorder. Seek a knowledgeable practitioner who can find the pieces of the puzzle and put them back together with targeted nutrient therapies.

"The time to relax is when you don't have time for it."
—*Sydney J. Harris*

You deserve to have energy, strength, restful sleep, motivation, joy, laughter, happiness, clear thinking, peace, healthy digestion, balanced hormones and a pain-free body.

Choose to live your best life. You deserve it.

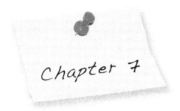

Chapter 7

DANCING PARTNERS: HORMONES, NEUROTRANSMITTERS, THYROID, ADRENALS

Have you ever seen a doctor who treated you with female hormones but you still didn't feel right? Perhaps you also had a thyroid imbalance, adrenal fatigue or a neurotransmitter deficiency.

All imbalances need to be treated.

In my practice, most women think of "hormones" as just estrogen, progesterone, and sometimes testosterone. Throughout a woman's lifetime she will experience fluctuating hormones and attribute mood swings, anxiety, depression, fatigue, joint pain, weight gain, low libido, hot flashes, cravings, mental confusion or memory loss, and insomnia to their imbalance. A woman's body is much more complex than just the sex hormones. Frequently, this is only one piece of the puzzle.

Often when a woman experiences premenstrual syndrome (PMS), perimenopause, or menopause, she is prescribed female hormones to relieve the symptoms. When this is not effective or symptoms remain, the hormones are changed or the dose is increased. Prescribing female hormones alone often does not result in the best outcome.

I have found that the common variety of menopausal symptoms may be due to a neurotransmitter imbalance, low thyroid, adrenal fatigue, toxins or a nutrient deficiency. The fluctuating levels of hormones such as estrogen, progesterone, testosterone, cortisol, and thyroid interact with brain neurotransmitters such as calming serotonin and GABA or excitatory dopamine, nor-epinephrine, epinephrine, glutamate, and others and cause a variety of symptoms.

I know this might sound complicated, but sometimes dances are. All these steps affect our emotional and physical responses to life, to stressors in our environment, to insults, and even to infections.

Neurotransmitters, which carry messages to every organ, muscle and gland, are affected by poor nutrition, medication, heavy metal toxicity, and overstimulation, which can impair the function of all systems. Thus, balancing our body's systems is a delicate dance, and one that requires many lessons and a lot of experience. It also requires a physician who is trained in the testing, diagnoses, and treatment of multiple bodily systems.

Functional medicine is a field of specialty that has a systems approach and treats the whole person.

Comprehensive and specialized testing can give you the blue prints to determine the root cause of these symptoms. Simply increasing the dose of the estrogen and progesterone may not be the answer to relieving the symptoms and may place women at a higher risk for multiple diseases. Finding the answers to your health is a process of putting together the pieces of the puzzle. When the deficiencies are resolved, toxins are removed and neurotransmitters, hormones and fatty acids are balanced, you will be on the journey to optimal health.

Since neurotransmitters affect hormones and hormones affect neurotransmitters, their imbalances can lead to increased symptoms and chronic illnesses. Taking preventive and proactive measures can ward off disease and suffering.

These dancing hormones and their interactions are responding not only to each other, but are modulated by our lifestyles and are significantly impacted by our stress. The complicated interaction of our hormones and our brain chemistry challenges our stress adaptation mechanisms, resulting in fatigue.

If you don't look and find the root cause of your symptoms, how do you really know what is wrong? Is your doctor testing all of your dancing hormones?

Doing the Menopausal Mambo

It is important to note that menopausal therapies include not only hormones, but mind/body support, exercise, good nutrition, appropriate supplements, self-care and laughter. The primary purpose is to manage the transitions, prolong life and preserve a healthy, active lifestyle. The approach to achieving these important goals is to *normalize* as many hormones as possible by using natural approaches and conventional pharmacology only when indicated.

Many health care practitioners have a limited understanding of all the therapeutic options for menopause symptoms and for the more global issues of menopause. Each woman wants to know if hormone replacement therapy is right for her, how she may benefit, how long she will have to undergo therapy to receive benefits, and if there are side effects or potential long-term risks.

The imbalances in the sex hormones create the following symptoms in women and men. These symptoms, however, may be related to other hormonal and neurotransmitter imbalances as well, which we will look at later in this chapter. What is the root cause of these symptoms? We may think that "we" have the answer. But the "answer" is complex and multi-faceted:

- **Mood swings:** Low serotonin, low thyroid, low GABA, high dopamine, low adrenals, low blood sugar, imbalanced EFAs (essential fatty acids).
- **Insomnia:** Low adrenals, low serotonin, low GABA, high NE (nor-epinephrine) , high EPI (epinephrine), low blood sugar, high cortisol, high thyroid, imbalanced EFAs.
- **Hot flashes:** High cortisol, low serotonin, and imbalanced EFAs.
- **Fatigue:** Low thyroid, low DHEA, low glutamate, low adrenals (cortisol), low dopamine, low NE, low EPI, and imbalanced EFAs.

- **Anxiety:** Low serotonin, low GABA, high NE, high EPI, high glutamate, high cortisol, and imbalanced EFAs.
- **Depression:** Low serotonin, low thyroid, low Vitamin D, low NE, high glutamate and imbalanced EFAs.
- **Pain:** Low serotonin, low vitamin D, low cortisol, high NE and imbalanced EFAs.
- **Lack of motivation:** Low serotonin, low dopamine and imbalanced EFAs.
- **Carbohydrate cravings:** Low serotonin, insulin resistance, low dopamine and imbalanced EFAs.
- **Weight gain:** Low thyroid, high cortisol, insulin resistance and imbalanced EFAs.
- **Memory loss and loss of focus:** Low thyroid, low cortisol, low dopamine, low EPI, low NE, low glutamate and imbalanced EFAs.
- **Decreased libido:** Low thyroid, low DHEA, low testosterone and imbalanced EFAs.
- **PMS:** Low serotonin, low dopamine and imbalanced EFAs.

The following graph shows that there are many reasons that cause the same symptoms:

Hormones	Food Allergies	Neurotransmitters
Anxiety	Anxiety	Anxiety
Depression	Depression	Depression
Insomnia	Insomnia	Insomnia
Fatigue	Fatigue	Fatigue
Joint ain	Joint Pain	Joint Pain
Memory Loss	Memory Loss	Memory Loss
Poor Concentration	Poor Concentration	Poor Concentration
Low Libido	Low Libido	Low Libido
Carb Cravings	Carb Cravings	Carb Cravings
Muscle Stiffness	Muscle Stiffness	Muscle Stiffness

Neurotransmitters

Neurotransmitters include the inhibitory serotonin and GABA, and excitatory nor-epinephrine (NE), epinephrine (EPI), glutamate, and dopamine. Neurotransmitter imbalances can cause a wide range of mental, physical, and emotional symptoms. For example, low levels of serotonin can cause anxiety, depression, and pain, lack of motivation, insomnia, and carbohydrate cravings.

If your neurotransmitters are not in balance, brain fog will occur. Low levels of dopamine, nor-epinephrine, epinephrine, or glutamate create lack of focus and low brain function. Once tested, the individual can be treated with specific amino acids to correct the imbalance for better brain function.

The brain needs to be fed. According to Dr. David Perlmutter, a well known nutrient-oriented neurologist, the single most important thing you can do to keep your brain functioning at its peak and prevent brain aging is what you put on your plate. It's as simple as that.[1]

Nutrition is the most important tool for staying mentally and physically fit, and is by far the most underutilized tool. When you think about it, the only way we live and heal is by the air we breathe, the water we drink and the food we eat.

The most important nutrient for your brain is fat. Yes, fat. *Fats is not a four letter word.* Sixty percent of our brain is made out of fat. The brain's 100 trillion cell walls are made up of 60–80 percent fat. Brain-friendly fats include those from seeds (hemp, sunflower, flax, chia, pumpkin), organic cold pressed oils from hemp, sunflower, safflower, chia, flax, egg yolk, organic butter, high quality fish oil and wild salmon, sardines, anchovies, generous amounts of balanced, and good fats/oils rich in essential fatty acids. Omega 3 and Omega 6 are the keys to optimal brain health.

Beware of trans-fats that are found in processed baked goods, condiments, processed and fried foods. They make rigid, tough, slow brain cells. *Keep these fats off your plate.*

Customized individual therapies, including therapeutic lifestyle changes, nutrition and supplements when indicated, can be tailored to correct the imbalances.

Do you have low thyroid?

The thyroid is a small, butterfly-shaped gland located in the front of the neck below the larynx, or voice box. The thyroid gland makes two thyroid hormones, triiodothyronine (T3) and thyroxine (T4), which circulates in the bloodstream and acts on virtually every tissue and cell in the body. Thyroid hormones affect metabolism, brain development, breathing, heart and nervous system functions, body temperature, muscle strength, skin dryness, menstrual cycles, weight, cholesterol levels, and more.

Hyperthyroidism and hypothyroidism are most often caused by autoimmune diseases. Graves disease causes a hyperactive thyroid while the end result of Hashimoto's thyroiditis is hypothyroidism or low thyroid function. So what causes autoimmune disease? One consideration is low stomach acid and the other is inflammation.

The "itis" is inflammation and it is coming from somewhere. In thyroid conditions and other inflammatory conditions it is important to find the root cause of the inflammation. So whether you have neuritis from the nerves or brain, sinusitis, gastroenteritis, arthritis, myositis (inflamed muscles), or any other "itis", it is coming from some underlying cause.

Is your doctor finding the underlying cause of your inflammation?

Signs of Low Thyroid

There are a variety of signs and symptoms of low thyroid function. Maybe you have had your thyroid tested and it is "normal." Many times hypothyroidism (low thyroid function) is misdiagnosed.

In addition to the symptoms indicated on the following page, another sign can be elevated cholesterol (generally seen as elevated LDL cholesterol), fibromyalgia and easy bruising.

I can personally attest to the relationship of low thyroid and high cholesterol as I was diagnosed with high cholesterol with no apparent reason or risk factors. My thyroid levels were borderline low and my doctor didn't think it was necessary to treat the lower thyroid function because my numbers, although low, were in the reference range "box." When I persisted and was placed on thyroid medication, my cholesterol dropped 50 points without any other changes. Thyroid burns fat, especially very long chain fatty acids that can build up in our cells after exposure to toxins and cause inflammatory and cellular structural abnormities/function.

If you experience the following symptoms, you may have low thyroid function:

• fatigue	• joint pain and swelling
• weight gain	• muscle cramps
• constipation	• irritability
• fuzzy thinking	• memory loss
• low blood pressure	• abnormal menstrual cycles
• fluid retention	• decreased libido
• body pain	• slow reflexes
• weakness	• depression
• dry, pale skin	• hair loss and dry hair
• cold intolerance	• loss of outermost eyebrows

According to the President of the American Association of Clinical Endocrinologist (AACE), Richard A. Dickey, MD, "Patients who have been diagnosed with high cholesterol should ask their physician about having their thyroid checked. If they have an underlying thyroid condition in addition to their high cholesterol, the cholesterol problem will be difficult to control until normal levels of thyroid hormone are restored."[2]

Fewer than half of the adults diagnosed with high cholesterol know if they have ever been tested for thyroid disease, despite the well-documented connection between the two conditions. The National Institutes of Health (NIH)[3] and the Food and Drug Administration (FDA) both recommend thyroid testing in patients with high cholesterol levels. The prescribing information for the popular cholesterol-lowering drugs also recommends that patients be tested for thyroid disease before beginning cholesterol-lowering drug therapy.

In healthy people, the thyroid makes just the right amounts of two hormones, T4 and T3, which have important actions throughout the body. These hormones regulate many aspects of our metabolism, eventually affecting how many calories we burn, how warm we feel, and how much we weigh. In short, the thyroid "runs" our metabolism.

These hormones also have direct effects on most organs, including the heart which beats faster and harder under the influence of thyroid hormones. Optimal thyroid function affects every cell in our body. On a cellular level, there can be no optimal nutrition absorption, detoxification of wastes or stimulation of oxygen consumption without adequate thyroid balance. T3, the active thyroid hormone, is created from T4 in the liver, so a healthy liver is important.

The first step to attaining the correct information is testing your TSH level, and thyroid levels such as free T4 and free T3, reverse T3 and thyroid antibodies. Keep in mind that a doctor telling you that your TSH is "fine" is not enough, because if your doctor is using the old standard normal range of 0.5 to 5.0, you could have a TSH of 4 and be told that you are "normal." In fact, your thyroid is not functioning adequately.

Many doctors today are following the new, recommended TSH range of 0.3 to 2.50. Free T4 and free T3 should be in the mid-range of the reference levels instead of the low-end for optimal thyroid function. Thyroid auto anti-antibodies (antibodies directed against the thyroid gland) are important to measure and evaluate in order to obtain balance.

Don't just settle for a TSH test. That is not enough to give you the answers you need to evaluate your thyroid. About 30 million women and 15 million men have this common medical condition.[4]

Causes of Low Thyroid

Psychosocial, chemical and physical stressors lower levels of T3, the active thyroid hormone.

One of the most important factors that lead to hypothyroidism is exposure to environmental toxins. Pesticides, mercury and stress are factors in causing thyroid dysfunction. Inflammation also creates or exacerbates all illnesses—the thyroid is no exception. Gluten sensitivity is directly related to auto-immune disease and may be a cause of Hashimoto's thyroiditis.

Nutrient deficiencies are other causes. Vitamin A, zinc, Essential Fatty Acid, for example, act to improve T3 binding in your cells. Iodine is the central ingredient in thyroid hormones T3 and T4. Iodine is an essential element that enables the thyroid gland to produce thyroid hormones. The body does not make iodine, so it is an essential part of your diet. Trying to produce T3 and T4 without iodine is like trying to swim without water.

Selenium is a component of the enzyme that helps convert T4 to T3, so deficiencies of selenium may impair thyroid function and promote hypothyroidism. Brazil nuts are naturally high in selenium, thus having one daily serving will supply selenium needs with a natural food source.

In the United States, the most common cause of hypothyroidism is Hashimoto's thyroiditis, a condition that causes the body's defenses—the immune system—to produce antibodies that over time destroy thyroid tissue. As a result, the thyroid gland cannot make enough thyroid hormone. Researchers studying Hashimoto's thyroiditis have found that treatment with the thyroid hormone replacement drug levothyroxine (LT4) can reduce the incidence of Hashimoto's thyroiditis, as well as help alleviate the symptoms of the disease even if the patient's thyroid function is normal at the time.[5]

Other less common causes of hypothyroidism include:

- Thyroid surgery
- Radioactive iodine therapy
- External beam radiation, which is used to treat some cancers, such as Hodgkin's lymphoma
- Infections
- Medicines: Lithium carbonate is one of the most common medicines
- Disorders of the pituitary gland or the hypothalamus
- Congenital hypothyroidism
- Pregnancy: About 2 percent of pregnant women in the United States get hypothyroidism

Therapy for Low Thyroid
- Identify sources of inflammation—usually pasta, bread, desserts (gluten /wheat and other grains), sweet fruits like grapes/dried fruit and sources of sugar in the diet

- Eat nutritious, low carbohydrate foods with high nutrient dense foods—seeds, nuts, green vegetables, berries, protein (meat, poultry, fish, legumes, eggs, goat milk feta cheese), cold pressed, organic oils
- Have the complete thyroid panel retested one month after initiating therapy

Once placed on thyroid medication, an important step is to determine if you are on the right drug. The majority of thyroid patients start out with levothyroxine, a synthetic T4 drug, usually the Synthroid brand. But if you are not feeling well on Synthroid, or another brand you are taking, you may want to ask your doctor about trying a different brand. The brands all have different fillers and binding ingredients and some are more easily dissolved or absorbed than others, so some people find they do better on one brand versus another.

Common natural brand names include Armour Thyroid and Nature-Throid. These are FDA-regulated, prescription drugs—not to be confused with over-the-counter, non-prescription thyroid glandulars available at the vitamin store. Both Nature-Throid and Armour Thyroid are a type of hormone that differs from other replacement therapy in that it provides both of the key thyroid hormones levothyroxine (T4) and L-triiodothyronine (T3).

For some people, even if the TSH level is normal, one may be functionally hypothyroid due to the body's inability to convert circulating T4 thyroid hormone into the active T3 hormone at the cellular level.

Patients may find that adding T3, in the form of Cytomel or via a compounded, time-released T3, to their levothyroxine (T4), resolves symptoms. Others seem to feel best on the natural desiccated T4/T3 drug Armour Thyroid or Natur -Throid which has been available by prescription for more than 100 years.

Can you head down to the local health food store, pick up some supplements, make a few dietary changes and fix your thyroid problem yourself? Probably not. Your thyroid hormonal balance is complex. Thyroid hormone is related to and interacts with many other hormones and neurotransmitters.

High levels of cortisol and inflammatory markers have been associated with decreased thyroid function. High levels of cortisol (which can also be caused by high stress levels, low testosterone, etc.) can directly lead to suppression of pituitary TSH secretion, and impair conversion of T4 to T3, and can impair serotonin function.

Thyroid function and serotonin activity are highly linked. In hypothyroidism, serotonin production is reduced. Adequate serotonin production is necessary to maintain thyroid hormone levels. Both need to be addressed in order to optimize function.

You may have heard that foods in the Brassica family such as cabbage, brussel sprouts, broccoli, and cauliflower affect thyroid function. These studies have been done on animals and at higher amounts than we get in a normal diet. Human studies provide no clear evidence that normal intake of these foods induces thyroid abnormalities.[6]

Treating thyroid alone without balancing other hormones often results in less than optimal results. Appropriate treatment can prevent the condition from progressing and prevent more weight gain and atherosclerosis along the way. Untreated or under-treated hypothyroidism can cause infertility, endanger pregnancy, or cause other hormonal problems, such as erratic menstrual cycles or difficult menopause.

Nutrients required for T4 manufacture include:

- Iodine
- Zinc
- Vitamins A, E, B2, B3, B6, and C
- Nutrients required to convert T4 to the more active T3 are zinc and selenium

Here are some things to consider:

1. If you have symptoms suggestive of hypothyroidism, see a doctor who can perform a comprehensive assessment and order appropriate labs to evaluate your thyroid hormones.
2. Test neurotransmitters, cortisol, sex hormones, red cell fatty acids, iodine, zinc and selenium.
3. Eat healthy foods to support thyroid health—preferably organic.

4. Decrease your stress. Cortisol will be lower and your thyroid health will be better!

5. Enjoy life! It supports serotonin, the happy calming neurotransmitter which supports thyroid!

Adrenal Hormones

Another partner with the dancing hormone is the adrenal hormones. The adrenal glands reside just above the kidneys. Sometimes they are called kidney caps, because it looks like the kidneys have little hats on them. The name Adrenal literarily means: ***Ad*** = at or near ***Renes*** = kidneys. So the name is telling us the position of the adrenal glands in the human body.

Do you find yourself saying things like, "Help, I want to feel better!"?

Do you feel tired, suffer from lack of sleep, and have joint pain or muscle stiffness, frequently catch the flu or colds, feel anxious and depressed, and have headaches or gastrointestinal disturbances, difficulty concentrating or remembering, or experiencing various allergy symptoms?

Do you have difficulty getting up in the morning, more fatigue from 3:00–5:00 PM, and get a second wind in the evening? Are you craving salt? Do you feel lightheaded? Are you sensitive to loud noises? Do you or others see you as "not your old self?"

My patients tell me they have seen a physician and all the tests were "normal" but they know they don't feel well. You may have seen your physician who ordered a panel of labs. Most fatigues don't show up on our annual physical.

The labs were normal and your physician says, "You're fine." But you know you are tired and lack energy. Some days you're so low on energy that you're drowsy by lunchtime and in need of a nap by mid-afternoon. What's making you so tired all the time? Stress, poor eating habits, overwork, even medical treatments can wear you down and cause fatigue.

Some of my patients were told by well-meaning doctors, "you are too stressed or too busy." You may actually have a blood chemistry imbalance and you may have adrenal fatigue. If this sounds all too familiar, you are not alone. Here is Jean's story.

I came to Doctor Norling, suffering from Chronic Fatigue. Although my routine lab work from conventional doctors showed nothing was wrong, I felt that I needed to take charge of my own heath and find out what was causing me to feel so terrible. Dr. Norling's specialized testing uncovered <u>plenty</u> of hidden causes of my symptoms—some minor, but some more serious. The neurotransmitter, gastrointestinal DNA, and the Acumen lab tests were truly eye opening for me.

I was thrilled to have found a doctor that was more focused on finding the source of my problems, not just giving me a pharmaceutical band-aid for my symptoms. Dr. Norling's IV treatments and natural supplements were successful in helping me to regain my energy and my overall health.

I was originally hesitant to use a doctor outside my network. I now realize it was the best move I could have made for my health and wellbeing. Dr. Norling took the steps to learn specifically how MY body works, and how to best approach MY path to healing. Her time and attention to my health has given me my own "roadmap" for health, which is priceless.

What is adrenal fatigue, how do you diagnose it, and what are the solutions? Eighty percent of people will suffer adrenal fatigue at some point in their lives, says Dr. James Wilson, author of the best-selling book *Adrenal Fatigue: 21st Century Stress Syndrome.*[7] Adrenal fatigue affects women primarily, yet it has been dismissed and largely untreated by the medical community.

Adrenal fatigue has a broad spectrum of non-specific yet often debilitating symptoms; the most common is feeling physically run down and emotionally spent. The onset of this disease is often slow and insidious. Patients are told that they are stressed and need to learn to relax more. But there is more to the story.

Adrenal fatigue can wreak havoc with your life. In the more serious cases, the activity of the adrenal glands is so diminished that you may have difficulty getting out of bed for more than a few hours per day. Individuals with adrenal fatigue often have difficulty getting up in the morning no matter how long they have slept! With each increment of reduction in adrenal function, every organ and system in your body is more profoundly affected. Changes occur in your carbohydrate, protein and fat metabolism, fluid and electrolyte balance, heart and cardiovascular system, and even sex drive. Your body does its best to make up for under-functioning adrenal glands, but it does so at a price.

Today, adrenal fatigue can be accurately diagnosed and overcome by specific natural approaches. According to a study from the *American Psychological Association*, 2007:[8]

- 33 percent of Americans feel they are living with extreme stress.
- 75 percent say that money and work are the leading causes of stress.
- 48 percent feel that their stress has increased over the past five years.

Once your brain senses some kind of stress, your heart begins to race, you become hyper vigilant, and mentally alert. Your body's central nervous system has switched to fight-or-flight mode. The adrenal glands pump out epinephrine, cortisol, and other hormones that affect your heart, lungs, circulation, metabolism, and immune system.

Heart rate and blood pressure increase bringing more blood to your muscles and brain (to make split-second decisions). Blood sugar rises to increase fuel for energy, and the blood clotting ability also increases to survive injuries. This is an important emergency function of the body to be used sparingly. When the adrenal glands activate hormones to meet a stress response daily or weekly, the adrenals become depleted and your health is at risk.

Women wonder why they don't recover as quickly as they used to. Their body becomes adapted to the stress in their lives and they are not as able to bounce back. The most common causes of stress are work pressure, financial worries, death of a loved one, moving homes, changing jobs, illness, marital disruptions and concerns about children. I knew a woman who was faced with all these at the same time.

Prolonged periods of high stress, imbalanced lifestyle (lack of sleep, too little exercise and poor nutrition), and frequent physical exhaustion stress the adrenals. As a result, adrenal fatigue occurs—the amount of stress overextends the capacity of the body to compensate and recover from stress.

The late Hans Selye, MD,—Professor and Director of the Institute of Experimental Medicine and Surgery at the University of Montreal and known as the "Father of Stress" first described the general adaptation syndrome in 1945. These are the four stages of adrenal fatigue.[9]

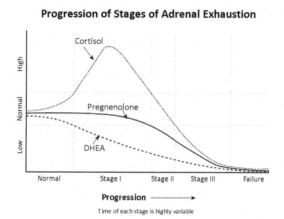

as the "Father of Stress" first described the general adaptation syndrome in 1945. These are the four stages of adrenal fatigue.

Progression of Stages of Adrenal Exhaustion

Stage One: Adrenal Stress

At this time, you may feel tired or wired and anxious or both. You may have trouble falling asleep, have a depressed immune system, experience headaches, aches and pains and gastrointestinal symptoms.

Stage Two: Adaptation

If your stress continues, your body may adapt to it like it is normal. Your body may not be noticing the elevation of hormones such as cortisol, insulin, nor-epinephrine and epinephrine. This is a false sense of security. During this period, the body needs cortisol to overcome stress, and production of cortisol is increased leading to obesity, diabetes and other illnesses. Over time, the adrenals will be unable to meet the body's ever increasing demand for cortisol and will become depleted.

Stage Three: Adrenal Exhaustion

As the stress continues unabated, the first symptoms return with a vengeance. Other symptoms and illnesses begin to occur. The body loses its ability to cope and resist the stimuli it once handled with ease. You may develop allergies you never had before or get sick over and over again. Seemingly unrelated symptoms occur like increased fatigue, low libido, insomnia, PMS or menopausal symptoms, anxiety or irritability, heart palpitations, high blood pressure, weight gain, and more severe heartburn, brain fog or irritable bowel syndrome.

Severe sex hormone imbalances (estrogen, progesterone, and androgens) are common and a precursor to adrenal failure. Total cortisol output is therefore reduced, and DHEA falls far below average.

Hormones all have a relationship to each other. They react to the levels of other hormones as they adjust to the needs of the body. When adrenal fatigue occurs in women the signs and symptoms are often confused with PMS or menopausal symptoms. It is important for women to work with a physician who can help her sort out the hormone dilemma.

Stage Four: Physical Decline

Eventually your body's ability to resist or adapt is compromised—symptoms occur and the old symptoms increase in severity. Women are completely exhausted and may fall asleep easily, but wake up during the night and have problems getting back to sleep. In this stage we see all sorts of chronic illnesses like depression, low blood sugar, GERD and colitis.

If you have a genetic predisposition to any type of autoimmune disease or a severe disease, the adrenal fatigue may trigger its onset at this time. These diseases can include rheumatoid arthritis, fibromyalgia, heart disease, multiple sclerosis, osteoporosis, cancer or diabetes.

Cortisol works with insulin from the pancreas to provide adequate glucose to the cells for energy. More energy is required when the body is under stress from any source, and cortisol is the hormone that makes this happens. With adrenal fatigue, more cortisol is secreted during the early stages increasing the risk of diabetes. In later stages (when the adrenal glands become exhausted), cortisol output is reduced, and blood sugar balance becomes a problem.

Cortisol is a powerful anti-inflammatory agent. Its objective is to remove and prevent swelling and redness of nearly all tissues. As cortisol is diminished an increase in inflammation is the result. People with high cortisol levels are much weaker from an immunological point of view. Cortisol influences most cells that participate in the immune system reaction and suppresses white blood cells, natural killer cells, monocots and macrophages, placing women at increased risk of infections and other diseases.

Cortisol contracts mid-size arteries. People with low cortisol (as in advance stages of adrenal fatigue) have low blood pressure. High cortisol tends to increase blood pressure that is moderated by calcium and magnesium. People with adrenal fatigue cannot tolerate stress and will then succumb to severe stress.

As their stress increases, progressively higher levels of cortisol are required. When the cortisol level cannot rise in response to stress, it is impossible to maintain the body in optimum stress response and an increase in symptoms and a decline in overall health occurs. Your body is crying out for help and attention.

Adrenal fatigue should not be confused with another medical condition called Addison's disease where the adrenal glands are not functioning. While Addison's disease is often caused by auto-immune dysfunction, adrenal fatigue is caused by stress. Adrenal fatigue afflicts more people than Addison's disease. Adrenal fatigue clearly is not properly recognized and diagnosed and, as a result, has become an epidemic of massive proportion in our society. To truly diagnose adrenal fatigue, more sensitive specialized laboratory testing and meticulous review of the medical history is required. Is your doctor using the right specialized testing for adrenal fatigue?

Is your doctor using the right specialized testing for adrenal fatigue?

Successful treatment of hormone imbalances requires looking beyond the sex hormones, neurotransmitters and thyroid system. Properly diagnosing and treating adrenal fatigue is an important piece of the puzzle. When adrenals are stressed, estradiol can be shunted to DHEA, testosterone to DHEA, and progesterone to cortisol.

In menopausal women, the adrenal glands are the only source of DHEA. In menopausal woman, the adrenals are the only source of testosterone, and they produce estrogen and progesterone. If the adrenals are exhausted and cortisol is low, menopausal and PMS symptoms intensify. Adrenal evaluation and normalization should precede hormone therapy.

Addressing the overall health of the adrenal function, neurotransmitters, and thyroid function is more effective in the long run than the Band-Aid approach of replacing deficient hormones alone. Measuring and treating only one system is a misguided practice. The communication system is complex and symptoms overlap.

Your treatment using natural approaches, including specifically designed supplements with the building blocks of the hormones and neurotransmitters, can then be tailored to your individual needs.

All the dancing hormones need to be evaluated and treated as indicated. Otherwise it is like standing on a one legged stool.

What's the solution?

- Decrease your stress by setting boundaries, delegating and just saying "no".
- Live a healthy lifestyle with good nutrition eating 6 times a day, exercise and sleeping 8 hours a night.
- Have your doctor order an adrenal test. One blood draw will not give you the information you need. You need to use an FDA lab that test your saliva four times in one day as the normal levels of cortisol fluctuate throughout the day. You may be normal at noon but high or low in the morning, evening and night. One blood test will not give your physician the needed information in order to balance your daily adrenal function.
- Adrenal fatigue can be treated successfully with specific targeted nutrient therapies, generous source of arachidonic acid found in egg yolk, organic butter, meat fat and goat cheese/goat milk feta.
- Consider acupuncture or craniosacral therapy to address the stress your adrenal fatigue.
- Get more pleasure from life. Have fun. Do the things you love. Get out in nature. Most importantly take time for yourself.

This is not pampering—this is good health.

Chapter 8

ADDICTIONS: RIGHTING THE WRONG

The time has come to recognize that addiction is no longer to be pushed into the dark corners and stigmatize the people that suffer from the disease.

Addiction has many faces: sex, gambling, drugs, and alcohol, to name a few. Sexual addiction is like any other addiction—it is destructive and painful to the addict's partner, the addict, as well as to their friends and family.

We joke about our addiction to chocolate and to shopping, but addiction is an intensely private, personal and confronting affliction that is as difficult to explain as it is to treat. This is a complex issue, but we know it is much more complicated than just drawing on willpower.

We have all been impacted at one time or another by addiction either personally or professionally. Maybe it is someone you know, a co-worker, a loved one, or … you. Addiction is an equal-opportunity affliction, affecting people without regard to their economic circumstance, education, race, geography, IQ or any other psycho-social factor. Many of today's addicts are educated, well-respected individuals such as executives, CEOs, doctors, lawyers, business people, housewives and their beloved family members.

No single factor determines whether or not a person will become addicted to drugs. Scientists estimate that genetic factors account for 40 to 60 percent of a person's vulnerability to addiction, including the effects of environment on gene expression and function.[1] Just because an individual has a family history of substance abuse does not mean that the gene needs to be expressed (activated). Genes are like light switches—they can be turned on and they can be turned off. However, the vulnerability increases with the environmental, social and biochemical, or neurotransmitter imbalances. Alcohol and drugs are just a quick and easy way to change ordinary, everyday reality from unbearable to bearable.

It is probably a confluence of factors, a potent but unknowable combination of nature and nurture that may or may not lead to addiction. Addiction and alcoholism are only symptoms of a deeper underlying cause.

- According to the Substance Abuse and Mental Health Services Administration's (SAMHSA's) National Survey on Drug Use and Health[2], 23.5 million persons aged 12 or older needed treatment for an illicit drug or alcohol abuse problem in 2009 (9.3 percent of persons aged 12 or older). Of these, only 2.6 million—11.2 percent of those who needed treatment received it at a specialty facility.

- SAMHSA also reports characteristics of admissions and discharges from substance abuse treatment facilities* in its Treatment Episode Data Set http://www.drugabuse.gov/publications/drugfacts/treatment-statistics—sources (TEDS).

- According to TEDS, there were 1.8 million admissions in 2008 for treatment of alcohol and drug abuse to facilities that report to State administrative data systems.

- Most treatment admissions (41.4 percent) involved alcohol abuse. Heroin and other opiates accounted for the largest percentage of drug-related admissions (20.0 percent), followed by marijuana (17.0 percent).

Addiction and Risky Substance Use

The facts show that addiction and risky use are causal and contributing factors in more than 70 other conditions requiring medical care and drive a wide range of costly social consequences.

Data from Columbia University in 2012 shows that 40.3 million more people have addictions than have heart conditions (27.0 million), diabetes (25.8 million) or cancer (19.4 million). More than 20 percent of deaths are attributable to tobacco, alcohol, and other drug use. Risky users account for 80.4 million individuals who engage in the use of addictive substances in ways that threaten health and safety.[3]

According to the National Center on Addiction and Substance Abuse at Columbia University, the vast majority of addicts (96.5 percent) start their first substance use before age 21 when the brain is still developing. Unfortunately, 95.6 cents of every dollar spent by federal, state, and local governments on risky substance use and addiction go to pay for the consequences; only 1.9 cents go to prevention and treatment.[4]

Every year, abuse of illicit drugs and alcohol contributes to the death of more than 100,000 Americans. The consequences of drug and alcohol abuse are vast and varied and affect people of all ages. The consequences are medical, social, economic and criminal.

Surprisingly, prescription medications are increasingly being abused or used for non-medical purposes. This practice not only leads to addiction, but in some cases has a lethal outcome. Commonly abused classes of prescription drugs include painkillers, sedatives and stimulants.

Among the most disturbing aspects of this emerging trend is its prevalence among teenagers and young adults. Nearly one in 12 high school seniors report non-medical use of Vicodin® according to the NIDA's report (December 2011). Many people mistakenly believe that these medications are safe, even when used illicitly, because they are prescribed by physicians. They are not.

A recent study in Florida published in 2008 found that three times as many people were killed by legal drugs as by cocaine, heroin and all methamphetamines put together. In Florida in 2007, cocaine was responsible for 955 deaths, heroin for 121, methamphetamines for 25 and marijuana for zero, for a total of 989 deaths. In contrast, 2,328 people were killed by opioid painkillers, including Vicodin® and Oxycontin® and 743 were killed by drugs containing benzodiazepine, including the depressants Valium® and Xanax®. In 2005, 5.5 percent of high school seniors were using Oxycontin®. The facts are that these are just the reported cases. This may only represent a fraction of the true number of deaths by drugs.[5]

The Science of it all

Throughout much of the past century, scientists studying drug abuse labored in the shadows of powerful myths and misconceptions about the nature of addiction.

When science began to study addictive behavior in the 1930s, people addicted to drugs were thought to be morally flawed and lacking in willpower. Those views shaped society's responses to drug abuse, treating it as a moral failing rather than a health problem, which led to an emphasis on punitive rather than preventive and therapeutic actions.

Today, thanks to science, our views and our responses to drug abuse have changed dramatically. Groundbreaking discoveries about the brain have revolutionized our understanding of drug addiction, enabling us to respond effectively to the problem. As a result, researchers and scientists continue to put the pieces of the puzzle together of this complex disease.

Many well-meaning family members and friends will sometimes tell the addict basically to just have will power, a positive attitude, and stop using. We don't tell the diabetic to just have will power, a positive attitude, and stop using insulin. Just as there is a biochemical imbalance in the diabetic, there is one in the addict. While the positive attitudes and 12-step programs are a life saver for many, the biochemical neurotransmitters cannot be ignored.

Addiction is defined as a chronic, relapsing brain disease that is characterized by compulsive drug-seeking and use, despite harmful consequences. It is considered to be a brain disease because drugs change the brain; they change its structure and how it works. This is also true of pharmaceutical drugs that are prescribed for addicts. These brain changes can be long lasting, and can lead to the harmful behaviors seen in people who abuse drugs. Why use one addictive drug to replace another drug when other effective options are available?

Is it really a "disease"? Can it be cured? Is relapse inevitable?

Relapse is not inevitable. The brain has plasticity and can be healed. The one thing becoming clearer is that addiction not only has psychological, social, environmental and genetic components, but also biochemical imbalances.

The biochemical imbalances may precipitate in self-medicating with drugs and alcohol. Dr. Nora Volkow, the director of the NIDA was interviewed by the *Washington Post* in August of 2003, and stated the following; "I've studied alcohol, cocaine, methamphetamine, heroin, marijuana and more recently, obesity. There's a pattern in compulsion. I've never come across a single person that was addicted that wanted to be addicted. Something has happened in their brains that has led them to that process."

It is fundamental to the recovery process that the underlying cause(s) of the addiction be identified and treated

As a result of scientific research, we now know that addiction is a disease or a biochemical imbalance that affects both brain and behavior. We have identified many of the biological and environmental factors and are beginning to search for the genetic variations that contribute to the development and progression of the disease. Scientists use this knowledge to develop effective prevention and treatment approaches that can reduce the toll drug abuse takes on individuals, families and communities.

Brain Effects

Dopamine is a neurotransmitter present in regions of the brain that regulate movement, emotion, cognition, motivation and feelings of pleasure. *All drugs of abuse target the brain's reward system by increasing dopamine.* The over-stimulation of this system, which rewards our natural behaviors, produces the euphoric effects sought by people who abuse drugs and teaches them to repeat the behavior. When some drugs of abuse are taken, they can release two to 10 times the amount of dopamine that natural rewards do. The effect of such a powerful reward strongly motivates people to take drugs again and again.

Unfortunately, for every artificial drug-induced "high" (ex: psychoactive drug-induced mania), there is also a predictable and inevitable "crash" that results in the individual feeling artificially "low" (psychoactive drug-withdrawal depression or fatigue). People with drug-induced highs and lows or other drug-induced behaviors can easily be misdiagnosed as having a mental illness such as depression, anxiety, mania, bipolar disorder or psychotic disorder to name a few.

Over time the drug use depletes the brain of dopamine and the ability to produce it naturally. Inadequate levels of dopamine create lack of motivation and focus, cravings, and low libido—thus experiencing any pleasure is reduced.

This is why the abuser eventually feels flat, lifeless and depressed, and is unable to enjoy things that previously brought them pleasure. Now, they need to take drugs just to bring their dopamine function back up to normal. Meth users can deplete as much as 90 percent of their brain's dopamine. Chronic exposure to drugs of abuse disrupts the way critical brain structures interact to control behavior—behavior specifically related to drug abuse.

As the addict uses more, the neurotransmitters become deficient; lowering the levels of serotonin causes cravings, lack of motivation, pain, insomnia, anxiety and depression. Deficient levels of GABA cause anxiety, restlessness, insomnia, and excess worry. Low levels of glutamate cause low brain function and fatigue. All these conditions can make a person more vulnerable to seek sex, medications, drugs or alcohol to relieve their symptoms. Everyone wants to feel better.

Deficiencies or elevations of many specific neurotransmitters have a significant impact on mental, emotional and behavioral function. If the neurotransmitters are out of balance, the risk for addictions and relapse is much higher. Therefore, it makes perfect sense to test them when going into a recovery program.

Addiction is not a life sentence. When drug abuse takes over, a person's ability to exert self-control can become seriously impaired. Brain-imaging studies from drug-addicted individuals show physical changes in areas of the brain that are critical to judgment, decision making, learning and memory, and behavior control. The images change as the brain heals. The good news is that research shows the brain is plastic and it can be repaired! Brain images published in the *Journal of Neuroscience* in 2001 show the brain's remarkable ability to recover after prolonged substance abstinence. This is what is called *plasticity of the brain.*[6]

Physicians, family and community collectively ensure that the diabetic gets insulin so they don't relapse with high blood sugar due to insulin deficiency.

We test the blood sugar. When someone has low thyroid they are treated with thyroid replacement. But before we treat a thyroid problem we test thyroid function first.

How does one expect to avoid drug relapses unless neurotransmitters are tested and the nutrients that support neurotransmitters are replaced and balanced? The brain is 60 percent lipid.

We can test the red cell lipids at the Kennedy Krieger lab at Johns Hopkins and find gross suppression of the lipid content. The brain needs the structural and essential fatty acids to normalize. Labs are available to test nutrient deficiencies. The brain needs amino acids and vitamin co-factors to make neurotransmitters. Vitamin D3 levels should be tested—low levels of vitamin D3 can cause depression.

Addictions and Antidepressants

Did you know that psychiatrists are the only medical specialty that does not test the organ they treat—the brain? FDA neurotransmitter testing is readily available. Most doctors just prescribe without testing the neurotransmitters. Just writing a prescription for Zoloft®, Lexapro®, Celexa®, Wellbutrin®, Paxil®, Prozac®, or any mood-altering drug without neurotransmitter lab results can be a misguided practice.

Physicians also prescribe drugs like Methadone®, Suboxone® or Naltraxone®; essentially substituting one addictive drug for another. The fact is that antidepressants only temporarily increase the concentration of a neurotransmitter into the space between two nerves (while destroying some of the enzymes that feed the NT's at the same time); therefore resulting in long-term depletion within the secreting nerve cell.

Many people with addictions also suffer with mood disorders such as anxiety and depression.

- Approximately 8.9 million adults have co-occurring disorders; that is they have both a mental and substance use disorder.
- Only 7.4 percent of individuals receive treatment for both conditions with 55.8 percent receiving no treatment at all. According to the Substance Abuse and Mental Health Administration (SAMHSA).

- The brains of those who have been physically or sexually abused, psychologically or spiritually traumatized, neglected, isolated, labeled "mentally ill," experiencing psychiatric drug adverse effects or the temporary mental anguish of drug withdrawal may have the need to self-medicate their sadness, nervousness, nightmares, empty lives or the effects of their drugs.

In reality (and here is where the potential for cure exists), these individuals may not be able to produce enough of their essential neurotransmitters because of dietary deficiencies or the use of neurotransmitter-depleting drugs. People who experience the pain and suffering of mood disorders often turn to drugs to make them feel better. The neurotransmitter imbalances can be treated by targeted nutrient therapies. When the addict feels calmer, happier, well rested, focused and productive, the risk of relapse decreases.

The acute ingestion of alcohol (as well as many other prescription tranquilizers) temporarily and artificially increases the amount of calming neurotransmitters (ex: serotonin, GABA) into the synapses of certain brain nuclei.

Many of the drugs can be expected to cause a depletion of the very neurotransmitters that are required for the drugs to work! In addition, there is predictable, albeit unintended micro-anatomic (and eventually even macro-anatomic) brain damage that can occur with the chronic use of many types of psychoactive drugs, especially when used in high doses for a lengthy period of time or in combinations.

When the *Physician's Desk Reference* mentions neurologic or psychiatric side effects to a drug, you know it got to the brain from the blood stream. A peer-reviewed article authored by psychiatrist Peter R. Breggin in the *International Journal of Risk & Safety in Medicine* addresses this issue.[7]

Because of the reuptake pump inhibition mechanism of action of most drugs in the psycho-stimulant and antidepressant classes, we can predict why they stop working or cause dependencies, tolerance and withdrawal symptoms when tapered down or stopped abruptly.

Unfortunately, the way the brain was intended to work is seriously altered by the chronic over-stimulation (or suppression) of the receptor sites (or reuptake pumps) in the synapses because of the chemical tampering. This keeps the nerves from functioning normally by altering the normal manufacturing process, transportation, storage, release, recycling, and/or reuse of specific neurotransmitters.

Many patients testify to the fact that both psycho-stimulants and the so-called "Selective" Serotonin Reuptake Pump Inhibitors (SSRIs) give them a sense of feeling temporarily "better than well" (as long as they keep on taking the drug). Both classes of drugs have as their base structure—an amphetamine molecule (which consists of a benzene ring with an attached carbon side chain and any number of other chemical groups attached that affect how it works in the brain and body).

However, usually the feeling of improvement tends to diminish far too soon with the need to have the dose increased or a second or third drug added to maintain the effect or counter the inevitable adverse effects of the first drug.

The infamous psycho-stimulant drug cocaine and the other amphetamine-like drugs like Dexedrine®, Desoxyn® (Meth), Ecstasy®, Fen-Phen®, Ritalin® (methylphenidate), Adderall® (a cluster of amphetamines), Straterra®, Wellbutrin® and Vyvanse® all have benzene rings as their base molecule and so do all the second generation so-called SSRI "antidepressants" like Prozac®, Paxil®, Zoloft®, Luvox®, Celexa®, Lexapro®, Effexor® and Pristiq®.

What can be done about chronic drug use and addiction? That is the subject of a multi-billion dollar industry that is failing in its stated goals primarily because there is a lack of understanding of the anatomy and physiology of addiction and ignorance about brain nutrition. One of the basic problems is that the drug industry has consistently made false claims that their drugs are not addicting.

Many of my patients come to see me primarily because they knew they had become dependent on and addicted to their psych drugs which is epidemic. Their addictions are not just drugs or alcohol, the addiction can be sex.

Sexual Addiction

"He cheated on me," she said still in disbelief. "He cheated on me with someone I know, someone I worked with, and someone I had helped and supported. I loved him deeply and the shock and pain was excruciating."

As she continued her story, she shared that she thought they had a great marriage as did their family, friends and anyone who knew them as individuals or as a couple. "Why?" Was the question and "history" was the answer. He had cheated on all his ex-wives and ex-girlfriends. He was cheating on several all at the sametime. He admitted to multiple other affairs during their marriage.

According to the National Council on Sexual Addiction and Compulsivity, sexual addiction is defined as, "engaging in persistent and escalating patterns of sexual behavior acted out despite increasing negative consequences to self and others."

In addition to damaging the addict's emotional relationships, they put their partners at risk for physical injury, and sexually transmitted diseases.

The problem of sexual addiction often leads to feelings of guilt and shame. They also feel a lack of control over their behavior, despite negative consequences of the many facets of their lives such as financial, health, and their social environment.

According to Michael Herkov, PhD at PsychCentral, "Studies indicate that food, drug abuse and sexual interests share a common pathway within our brains' survival and reward systems. This pathway leads into the area of the brain responsible for our higher thinking, rational thought and judgment."[8]

"The brain tells the sex addict that having illicit sex is good the same way it tells others that food is good when they are hungry. These brain changes translate into a sex addict's preoccupation with sex and exclusion of other interests, compulsive sexual behavior despite negative consequences and failed attempts to limit or terminate sexual behavior."

Some of the known causes of being a sexual addict include:

Inconsistent parental nurturing and love and a sense of parental betrayal: the need to feel emotional love and support can make a person susceptible to turning to sex to find security.

Insufficient parental teaching and modeling: this can leave a child without a solid foundation of love and respect.

Early sexualization: sounds, sights and physical contacts that are inappropriate can cause a child to assign an improper place to sex in life.

All addictions have similar patterns. All addicts need to decide to end their addictions and make the choices necessary for recovery.

Where Does the Medical Profession Stand on Addictions?

According to National Center on Addiction and Substance Abuse, Columbia University.[10]

- 1956—AMA declared alcoholism an illness that can and should be treated within the medical profession.
- 1989—AMA adopted a policy declaring addiction involving other drugs, including nicotine, to be a disease.
- Research indicates 47 percent of Americans would turn to a health professional if someone close to them needed help for addiction. Yet less than six percent of referrals to publicly funded addiction programs come from a health care provider. Most come from the justice system.
- There are only about 1,200 practicing addiction medicine specialists and 355 self-identified practicing addiction psychiatrists out of 985,375 active physicians.
- Most treatment providers are addiction counselors—medical training is not required.
- 14 states do not require all addiction counselors to be licensed or certified.
- 6 states—no minimum degree requirements.
- 14 states—minimum requirement of High School Degree or GED.
- 10 states—minimum requirement of Associate's Degree.
- 6 states—minimum requirement of Bachelor's Degree.
- 1 state requires Masters Degree.

The public's attitude about addiction is out of sync with science. Center for Addiction and Substance Abuse at Columbia University's *NABAS* survey found that the public does not recognize the role of genetics and biological factors in the development of addiction. Of the respondents, 60 percent identified mutual support programs as "treatment" intervention.

Patients face formidable barriers to receiving addiction treatment due to misunderstanding of the disease, negative public attitudes and behavior toward those with the disease, and negative perceptions of the treatment process.[11]

The only thing stopping people from a new life is usually the ignorant actions and words of others and what they themselves would be labeled. Addiction is typically a chronic disorder characterized by relapses. For some, treatment can be a long term process that involves multiple interventions and regular monitoring. However, for many others it is the understanding of what led them to the use of drugs, alcohol or other addictions.

Addiction is a family problem and family therapy is critical. Family members suffer along with the addict in words that are difficult to describe. Many times the neurotransmitters of family members also have become imbalanced because of the stressors of having an addict in the family.

The key to recovery is not a simple program, of "one size fits all." Treating all addicts with the same therapies and treatments is overrated and many times unsuccessful. Successful recovery is greater in programs that are comprehensive, customized to the individual and where the addict is returned to an overall state of health. Some people respond better to individual counseling rather than group therapy sessions. A customized program is the key to success.

Addicts need to have the chance to regain their successful and happy life. Every life is a life worth saving. Here are some good starting points that addicts, their families, and friends should consider while looking for a program:

- Find a team of professionals that the addict and their family will resonate with that treats the whole person.
- Make sure the addict and their family receives support from certified therapists and counselors.
- See an integrative physician for accurate nutrient based testing and treatment.
- Have your neurotransmitters, general chemistry and red cell fatty acid tested from a university based laboratory.
- Balance neurotransmitters, chemistry and essential fatty acids using specific targeted nutrient therapy.

- Consider IV therapies to add nutrients and detoxify the body and that support brain function, (including intravenous phosphatidylcholine as Essentiale). IV therapy has 100 percent absorption with higher doses and is faster acting.
- Eat the right foods; No more sugar.
- Relax with meditation and yoga.
- Hypnotherapy to support recovery.
- Make time to address your spiritual needs.
- Enjoy the right exercise.
- Always stay educated about new ways of staying in recovery.

Never, ever give up hope for recovery—it can and does happen every day.

Chapter 9

HEART DISEASE: RIGHT SOLUTIONS

E ven though heart disease is the leading cause of death in the U.S., you have more influence in helping to prevent it than you think. Cholesterol levels (good-HDL and bad-LDL), essential fatty acid deficiencies/imbalances, high carbohydrate intake, stress, neurotransmitters, hormones, vitamin D, Coenzyme Q10 (CoQ10), even tea and chocolate all play important roles for controlling your heart health.

Coronary artery disease (CAD), one type of heart disease, is the leading cause of heart attacks. The most common cause of CAD is *atherosclerosis*, a condition that occurs when plaque builds in the arteries that supply blood to the heart. "About three-quarters of the population older than 30 years has some lesion related to atherosclerosis in the arterial tree. This lesion gets worse almost every day in all these people and will eventually result in closure of a vital artery in half of them, causing their death," said William P. Castelli, MD, director Framingham Heart Study.[1]

Preventing heart disease requires much more than simply screening for high cholesterol. Fifty percent of all people who experience a heart attack have normal cholesterol.

Inflammation

Cholesterol is not the problem. It is the inflammation which creates the plaques that causes atherosclerosis and heart disease. Heart disease, like so many other diseases, is caused primarily by inflammation. Diabetics have a higher risk of heart disease. Increased blood sugar and diabetes increase insulin levels. Insulin promotes inflammation which promotes cardiovascular disease (CVD), strokes and death.

Cardiovascular disease (CVD) is an inflammatory condition such as arthritis. A recent article published in *Arthritis & Rheumatism* noted, "… Overall, there was a 50 percent increased risk of death in patients with rheumatoid arthritis (RA). When looking at causes of specific deaths, patients with RA had a 59 percent increased risk of dying from ischemic heart disease (heart attack) compared with the general population and a 52 percent increased risk of death due to strokes."[2]

While statins have been shown to decrease the risk of death from heart disease, it may be due to their anti-inflammatory properties rather than the lowering of cholesterol. They inhibit nuclear factor kappa B (NF-KB). NF-KB is involved in inflammatory reactions, using EPA from fish oil, GLA from evening primrose oil, the short chain fatty acid butyrate and phosphatidylcholine and can accomplish the same anti-inflammatory effect naturally.

Could a hidden food allergy or an infection in your mouth or intestines be causing your heart disease? Find the root cause of your inflammation. The right test will help determine the cause of your inflammation.

Gastrointestinal disease

We know food allergies, gluten sensitivity, celiac disease and irritable bowel syndrome are all inflammatory diseases; therefore it should not come as a surprise that they, too, increase the risk of cardiac disease.[3] Gastrointestinal infections can also increase the risk of heart disease.[4] If you have risks for heart disease or have CVD, have your stool tested.

Toxins

Evidence-based medicine has clearly shown that clinicians must begin to pay more attention to some of the less-obvious factors that play a significant role in the development of obesity, diabetes, and CVD.

Blood lead levels as low as 5–9 ug/dL are associated with an increased risk from all causes, cardiovascular disease, and cancer. High levels of lead have been known to cause kidney and neurological impairment. However, these results from the National Health and Nutrition Examination Surveys (NHANES) study showed that low level of lead have significant health consequences.[5]

According to Menke, lead exposure, even as low as 2 mcg/dl is associated with a 55 percent increase in CVD, an 89 percent increase in heart attacks, and a 151 percent increase risk in strokes. It is estimated that 39 percent of the US population has serum levels in that range.[6]

Dr. Mark Houston, a cardiologist and Associate Clinical Professor of Medicine at Vanderbilt University Medical School presents the role of mercury toxicity in hypertension, cardiovascular disease and stroke. Mercury induces mitochondria (cellular powerhouses) dysfunction. The clinical problems associated with mercury toxicity also include the heart attacks, cardiac arrhythmias, atherosclerosis, and kidney problems.

Mercury can also increase serum and urinary epinephrine, nor-epinephrine, and dopamine. Specialized testing can determine your toxic load. Selenium and fish Omega-3 fatty acids antagonize mercury toxicity.[7]

If you don't test how would you find answers?

According to Dr. Houston, "Optimal nutrition, nutraceuticals, vitamins, antioxidants, minerals, weight loss, exercise, smoking cessation and moderate restriction of alcohol and caffeine in addition to other lifestyle modifications can prevent and control hypertension in many patients."[8] "Macronutrient and micronutrient deficiencies are very common in the general population, and may be even more common in patients with hypertension and cardiovascular disease due to genetic and environmental causes and prescription drug use."[9] Dr. Houston is the Director of the Hypertension Institute at Saint Thomas Hospital in Nashville, TN.

The bottom line is that metal toxins can cause CVD and increased mortality. Toxicity can be minimized. Toxins can be removed by specific

IV therapies, detoxifying foods, and supplements. Lifestyle changes can reverse CVD.

Plastics are everywhere in everything. Bisphenol A (BPA) is found in cans, plastic containers and plastic bottles. This is one reason you should never put plastic containers in the microwave or dishwasher. The heat tends to dissolve the plastic which provides an opportunity for us to be eating plastic-laden meals. Researchers have linked BPA to increased risk of CVD, diabetes, and liver problems.[10]

Other toxins have also been implicated. Polychlorinated biphenyls (PCBs) and chlorinated pesticides have been associated with increased risk of diabetes and cardiac problems.[11]

This is why you need to pay attention to your toxic exposure even if it is perceived to be a small amount. The dangers of low toxic exposures of any kind for any period of time can lead to a wide range of disorders.

Yet, in spite of the fact that toxins can increase CVD, the pharmaceutical companies and physicians focus on cholesterol like it was the only game in town! Does your cardiologist test for lead or mercury?

Stress

It is common knowledge that stress plays a major role in symptoms and illnesses. The relationship between stress, heart disease and sudden death has been recognized since antiquity.

The incidence of heart attacks and sudden death have been shown to increase significantly following the acute stress of natural disasters and more common in individuals subjected to chronic stress such as job stress. English physician William Harvey (1578—1657) wrote in 1628, "Every affection of the mind that is attended either with pain or pleasure, hope or fear, is the cause of an agitation whose influence extends to the heart."

One of the ways a man can decrease the risk of a heart attack is to have sex with his wife instead of his girlfriend. Scientists have warned that men who cheat on their wives have an increased risk of sudden death from cardiac arrest during sex. This is because they are often with younger women in unfamiliar settings, which adds extra stress. This revelation emerged from a report in the *Journal of Sexual Medicine*.[12]

Professor Glenn Levine, from Baylor College of Medicine in Houston, said autopsy reports of nearly 6,000 cases of sudden death found 0.6 percent happened during sex. Although a small proportion of the total, up to 93 percent of those who died during sex were thought to be engaging in extra-marital sex! [13]

Another recent study found in the *Journal of Sexual Medicine*, shows that unfaithful men risk not only their marriage but also their cardiac health, and sexual encounters away from home and with younger women are particularly dangerous. The precise reasons for the increase in heart attack death are still unclear, but researchers suggest that a guilty conscience, stress from keeping the affair a secret, and the stress of wining, dining and satisfying a woman who is likely to be younger than the man's wife could all contribute to the link. [14]

Neurotransmitters

Stress imbalances your neurotransmitters and an imbalance of neurotransmitters causes stress. Research frequently shows obesity, hypertension, anxiety, metabolic syndrome, and insulin-resistance are associated with high levels of nor-epinephrine, low epinephrine, and low cortisol.

Nor-epinephrine is an excitatory neurotransmitter creating stress, anxiety, pain, anger and high blood pressure. Elevations in epinephrine not only create stress and insomnia, but also increase blood sugar and insulin resistance. High cortisol can increase your abdominal girth and anxiety which can increase your risk for CVD.

Low epinephrine impacts lipids. Low cortisol which can cause adrenal fatigue can contribute to increased triglycerides and low levels of HDL-C, the good cholesterol. The bottom line is that your brain and your heart are connected—but we already knew that.

Get the right neurotransmitter test and use natural supplements without side effects whenever possible to achieve healthy brain balance.

Hormones

All hormones affect heart health. Look at the examples below:

- Low testosterone in men increases the risk of heart disease, high blood pressure, chest pain, diabetes, and arthritis.[15, 16, 17]
- Normal levels of testosterone can decrease cholesterol, increase bone and muscle mass, and increase libido. Testosterone also decreases inflammation, a common cause of CVD.[18]
- Testosterone decreases angina (chest) pain.[19] Normal testosterone levels in both men and women also result in more energy, a better sense of well-being, and less pain.
- Low thyroid can increase cholesterol and hypertension. Treating low thyroid can lower cholesterol. Always have your thyroid tests done checking your free T3, free T4 and TSH.

Bottom line: the right hormonal balance can help prevent heart disease.

Vitamin D

It is common knowledge that low Vitamin D has a significant increase for a variety of diseases. Yet, I am surprised that most of the patients that come to me have not been tested. If they have, many were told that their level is "normal" when the lab results were 20–40 ng/dl. The current recommended range is 50–70 ng/dl.

Even in sunny California 90 percent of my patients have low levels of vitamin D. Why? Because they are not out in the sun for 40 minutes a day with 40 percent of their body exposed. When they are in the sun they use sunscreen. While children are often low in vitamin D, the older we get the lower the ability for our skin to convert the UV rays into vitamin D.

Foods are not necessarily the best source of vitamin D. Fortified milk has only 100 international units (IU). Sardines and salmon are other foods that have vitamin D up to 300 IU. The new recommended daily amount of vitamin D is 1,000–2,000 IU. Vitamin D is a fat soluble vitamin so take your supplement with meals for better absorption.

If your levels of vitamin D are too low, a new study suggests that you may be at a significantly increased risk for stroke, heart disease and death. Researchers followed 27,686 people, aged 50 and older, with no history of cardiovascular disease. The participants were divided into three groups based on their vitamin D levels. After one year of follow-up, the researchers found that those with very low levels of vitamin D were 77 percent more likely to die, 45 percent more likely to develop coronary artery disease and 78 percent more likely to have a stroke, and twice as likely to develop heart failure compared to people with normal vitamin D levels.

"We concluded that among patients 50 years of age or older, even a moderate deficiency of vitamin D levels was associated with developing coronary artery disease, heart failure, stroke and death," said study co-author Heidi May, PhD, a cardiovascular clinical epidemiologist with the Intermountain Medical Center in Utah. She presented this study at the American Heart Association's annual meeting in 2010.[20]

The Framingham Heart Study followed 1,739 participants who had no CVD. The Framingham Heart Study is a long term, ongoing project that has conducted heart research since 1948. Researchers found those with low vitamin D had twice the risk of a heart attack, heart failure, or stroke over five years compared to those who had higher levels of vitamin D.[21]

The current optimal level is 60 ng per ml. Your lab results will help you decide if you should take 1,000 IU, 5,000 IU, 10,000 IU or for a short period of time 50,000 IU.

Has your doctor tested your 25(OH) D3 level to provide you with the right recommendations?

Statins

Statins are a widely used class of drugs. HMG-CoA reductase inhibitors (statins) are the best selling prescription drug class in the US, including Atorvastatin®, the best selling prescription drug in the world. [22, 23, 24] Statins need a closer look as they can cause life threatening adverse events (AE).

So why are they prescribed like they are the next best thing to sliced bread? And why does the FDA continue to approve drugs that are later recalled because of the serious and often deadly side effects?

This may be one reason; an analysis at the University of California at San Francisco of studies on "a heart drug" showed that 96 percent of authors with drug company ties showed it to be safe, compared to 37 percent of authors with no ties. *American Medical News,* Sept 2000.[25]

"The global cardiovascular therapeutic drug market was worth $140.7 billion in 2009, and is expected to grow by a compound annual growth rate (CAGR) of 2.7 percent to $144.5 billion in 2010.

"The hypertension segment recorded $64.9 billion in sales in 2009. By a large margin, hypertension is the largest segment within the cardiovascular market, driven by a large number of billion-dollar-plus therapies. The market is expected to grow to $65.3 billion in 2010.

"Treatment for hyperlipidemia recorded sales of more than $33 billion in 2009. Large therapeutic drugs including Lipitor® and Crestor® comprise a high concentration of this segment"[26]

Statins lower CoQ10 levels and inhibit a very important mevalonate pathway. Simply stated this pathway is responsible for normal metabolism. It is responsible for how our body works. It functions to make corticosteroids, sex steroids, bile acids, and vitamin D. When this pathway is disrupted we are at risk for hormonal imbalance, muscle pain and problems, and memory, mental and emotional changes.

Lowering CoQ10 is a long-overlooked but grave problem. In the *Archives of Neurology*, June 2004 research showed that after 14 days of using a statin, the levels of CoQ10 were significantly lower.[27]

Coenzyme Q10 (CoQ10) is a lipid-soluble antioxidant. CoQ10 is an essential cofactor in the mitochondria which are located in the cell and responsible for energy production. CoQ10 deficiency has been implicated in several clinical disorders including, but not limited to heart failure, hypertension, Parkinson's disease, and cancer. Patients can also experience muscle pain, difficulty walking and cardiomyopathy. Also documented are peripheral neuropathies, gastrointestinal symptoms, including liver injury and progression of cataracts.

A number of manifestations of skeletal muscular breakdown have been reported, including the most feared—rhabdomyolysis.

Adverse Events (AE) are side effects. They are dose-dependent, and risk is amplified by drug interactions that functionally increase statin potency, often through inhibition of the cytochrome P450 3A4 system.

An array of additional risk factors for statin AEs are those that amplify (or reflect) mitochondrial or metabolic vulnerability, such as metabolic syndrome factors, thyroid disease, and genetic mutations linked to mitochondrial dysfunction. This is important as the mitochondria function as the source of energy powerhouses in our cells. The mitochrondria affect every system and every function of our body.

Mitochondrial dysfunction may also underlie many non-muscle statin AEs. Evidence from RCTs and studies of other designs indicates existence of additional statin-associated AEs, such as cognitive loss, neuropathy, pancreatic and hepatic dysfunction, and sexual dysfunction.[28]

If you are taking a statin, be sure to talk to your doctor about taking CoQ10. The recommended amount varies between 60 mg twice a day and 300 mg twice a day. CoQ10 supplementation is essential for anyone who is taking a statin.

If you have high cholesterol, low HDL ("good" cholesterol), high LDL ("bad" cholesterol), and high triglycerides, what should you do?

Cholesterol

The National Institute of Health recommends that if you are diagnosed with high cholesterol you should follow a list of lifestyle changes for 12 weeks. Yes, that *is* their recommendation. Why? Because it is safe, effective and without side effects. If your cholesterol has not lowered after 3 months then consider using a statin.[29]

Lifestyle modification needs to remain the first line of therapy for cardiovascular disease and metabolic syndrome which includes hypertension, increased abdominal waist, increased blood sugar and triglycerides, and low HDL, the good cholesterol. Even if you are on a statin, it is still important to live a healthy lifestyle. Otherwise the next disease can be right around the corner.

A recent study conducted by Jennifer L. Jones, PhD, Robert H. Lerman MD, PhD, et al. in the *Journal of Clinical Lipidology* in 2011 stated that a Mediterranean-style and low-glycemic-load diet improved variables of metabolic syndrome in women, and an addition of phytochemical-rich medical food enhanced even more benefits.[30]

The medical food contained phytosterols, soy protein, and extracts from hops and acacia. After 12 weeks on the diet, there was a reduction of waist measurements, decreased blood pressure and triglycerides. In the group using the diet and medical food, additional improvements were also observed in lower plasma LDL, non-HDL cholesterol, apolipoprotein B concentrations, and apo B/apo A-I..

This natural approach was as equally or more effective than the data from statin use. And it does not shut down how the body works but supports it in healing itself. There are no side effects or adverse events and there are effective options to pharmaceutical drugs.

Why would you use a statin drug instead of other natural evidenced-based therapies?

Does your doctor give you options and recommend therapeutic lifestyle changes? This is really important for long term good health. It is also important to provide lifestyle support to the patients. Education empowers you.

The most important objectives in your armor against blood sludge and plaque are to:

- Clear your diet completely of processed oil (canola oil especially), margarine, hydrogenated vegetable oil, trans fat, commercial mayonnaise and salad dressing.
- Remove refined carbohydrates from your diet—sugar, white flour, processed food, pasta, bread, cookies, cake, muffins, pizza need to be dumped in the garbage. You will never control your high triglyceride level until you control your carbohydrate intake which includes not only sugar and white flour but soft drinks and sweetened yogurt.
- Optimize your diet with high amounts of green vegetables (cooked and as salads), berries, seeds, nuts, legumes, free range/wild meats (buffalo)/poultry/fish (sardines, anchovies, wild salmon), goat milk feta cheese, high intake of balanced essential fatty acids.
- Go nuts for health! Nuts are filled with good fats.

Supplement with heart healthy nutrients.

Unfortunately, most physicians do not follow these guidelines.

Most physicians reach for the prescription pad and write an order for a statin. Statins lower LDL. Yet a study published in the *American Heart Journal Circulation: Cardiovascular Quality and Outcomes*, January, 2009, found that nearly two-thirds of patients admitted to hospitals for heart attacks and cardiovascular events had low LDL-cholesterol levels, indicating they were not at high risk for heart problems.[31]

Statins may not be the right answer.

The millions of adults who currently use prescription statins to control their cholesterol levels may be inadvertently increasing their risk for developing age-related cataracts, new research suggests. After accounting for factors such as gender, cigarette use and high blood pressure, the team found that statin use was associated with a 57 percent increased risk for developing cataracts.

"The bottom line is that there appears to be an increased risk among people taking statins as far as getting cataracts," said study lead author, Elizabeth Irving, PhD., research chairwoman in the School of Optometry and Vision Science at the University of Waterloo in Ontario, Canada.[32]

The infamous Women's Health Initiative showed a relationship between statin use and the increased risk of diabetes in 48 percent of postmenopausal women. We know that diabetes increases the risk of cardiovascular disease. Sugar causes inflammation and inflammation is the cause of heart disease and most other chronic illnesses.[33]

Low cholesterol is not healthy!

Statins can also lower your cholesterol to a dangerously low level. Yet the pharmaceutical industry continues to recommend an array of cholesterol-lowering drugs while not mentioning the dangers of low cholesterol. Physicians continue to prescribe cholesterol-lowering drugs even though studies have shown an increased risk of cancer when the cholesterol is below 160 mg.

Unfortunately, the dangers of low cholesterol have not been well publicized. There is a wealth of articles and health books that discuss how to prevent high cholesterol, but very few on how to prevent or treat abnormally low cholesterol. At an international medical conference I attended in London in November 2010, speakers presented the data showing cholesterol below 160 was associated with doubling the risk of cancer.

In 1990, an NIH conference concluded from a meta-analysis of 19 studies that men and, to a lesser extent, women with a total serum cholesterol level below 160 mg (6th percentile) exhibited about a 10 to 20 percent **excess** total mortality compared with those with a cholesterol level between 160 to 199 mg. Low Cholesterol has been shown to increase the risk of dying from gastrointestinal and respiratory disease.[34]

Abnormally low levels of cholesterol may indicate:

- Hyperthyroidism, or an overactive thyroid gland
- Liver disease
- Inadequate absorption of nutrients in the intestines
- Malnutrition
- Poor metabolism
- Compromised health

Similarly, patients with environmental illness often have low cholesterol including those with sensitivity to foods, chemical or frequencies, like Wi-Fi. Infertility has also been linked to low cholesterol.

Cholesterol is essential for:

- Formation and maintenance of cell membranes (essential for life).
- Making hormones (progesterone, testosterone, estradiol, cortisol).
- Production of bile salts, which help to digest food.
- Conversion into vitamin D in the skin when exposed to sunlight.

Approximately one-third of the cholesterol is what we eat. Two-thirds of cholesterol is made by the liver. Very low cholesterol may mean your body is "shutting down" and not able to make its own cholesterol.

Cholesterol is not bad. Cholesterol makes up one-third of our cell membrane. It makes all our hormones. *Fats* is not a four letter word. Our brain is 60 percent fat. Like fats, our life and our health need balance. Good fats are one of the keys to optimal health.

Supplements

Research continues to document that good nutrition and appropriate supplements can improve health and decrease the risk of CVD, chronic illnesses and cancer. However, taking vitamins, minerals and other supplements orally may result in only about 35 to 40 percent absorption depending on the quality and stomach acid.

For preventing cardiovascular disease (CVD) and for your overall health, oral supplementations are paramount, but also consider intravenous (IV) nutritional therapies as an adjunct. The intravenous therapies are given in higher doses, work faster, and are 100 percent absorbed. Documented case studies have shown that using specific nutrient IV therapies such as phosphatidylcholine and phenylbutyrate can lower cholesterol significantly (100–185 mg in some cases), decrease LDL, and lower triglycerides.

What About Tea and Chocolate?

This research will definitely put a smile on your face.

Numerous studies have shown that cocoa has a protective effect against cardiovascular diseases. The reason for this has now been uncovered by researchers in Sweden. When a group of volunteers devoured a good-sized piece of 72 percent dark chocolate, it inhibited an enzyme in their bodies known to raise blood pressure. The findings, published in the *Journal of Cardiovascular Pharmacology*, were revealed by a group of drug researchers headed by Ingrid Persson.[35]

"We have previously shown that green tea inhibits the enzyme ACE, which is involved in the body's fluid balance and blood pressure regulation. Now we wanted to study the effect of cocoa, since the active substances catechins and procyanidines are related," says Persson. The study participants were between the ages of 20 and 45 and ate 75 grams of unsweetened chocolate.

The results showed a significant inhibition of ACE activity. The average was 18 percent lower activity than before the dose of cocoa, fully comparable to the effect of drugs that inhibit ACE and are used as a first-choice treatment for high blood pressure. So will dark chocolate in the future replace your ACE inhibitor for high blood pressure? It is a sweet thought.

The right facts about Heart Disease

- Approximately 16 million Americans have heart disease.
- Heart disease is the #1 cause of death in both men and women.
- 50 percent of men and 64 percent of women who experience sudden death had no previous symptoms.
- 68 percentof all heart attacks and strokes occur from clots, not from the narrowing of the arteries.
- One-third of all strokes affect individuals between 45 and 65 years of age.
- Cholesterol is not a reliable predictor of strokes.

An estimated 80 percent of patients who develop coronary artery disease have cholesterol levels comparable to those in healthy individuals, according to the *Jupiter Study* by the American Heart Association.[36]

Cholesterol is carried throughout the body in little balls called *lipoproteins*. It is the lipoproteins, not the cholesterol in them that leads to clogged arteries. Standard cholesterol testing provides only part of the picture, leaving many people with "normal" cholesterol numbers unaware that they are still at risk for a heart attack.

Prevention of heart disease really means "preventing" disease and should not be confused with early detection using the standard cardiovascular testing—EKG, treadmill, echo, vascular studies, angiography to name a few. While these tests are important they are "after the fact." Having a detailed lipoprotein particle profile specialty test gives you and your doctor the information needed to make effective treatment decisions to reduce your risk of heart disease and even a heart attack.

So how do you get the right lab(s) giving you the information to prevent CVD?

VAP Test

The VAP cholesterol test is recommended for comprehensive assessment of the risk for Coronary Artery Disease (CAD) and Metabolic Syndrome in "at-risk" patients. This recommendation rests on the inadequacy of the ordinary lipid panel to identify patients at risk for myocardial infarction,[37] and similarly, the inadequacy of fasting glucose and insulin testing to identify many patients with Metabolic Syndrome.[38]

The VAP cholesterol panel is commercially available, inexpensive and resolves the inaccuracy in today's calculated LDL values. Recently presented at the American College of Cardiology 2012, researchers Seth Martin, MD *et.al,* found that in 1.3 million patients, clinically significant misclassification of patients using the Friedewald formula (standard lipid panel) compared to direct measured VAP LDL by ultracentrifugation.[39]

The VAP identified LDL particles in a higher risk category. The VAP determines whether or not the LDL ("bad") cholesterol is large and buoyant or small and dense. Research results show that the large LDL sub-fractions were not associated with ischemic heart disease in men, but the smaller LDL increased the risk.

This evidence underscores the urgency of assessing patients with more advanced cardiovascular risk biomarkers than those included in standard lipid panels. Always ask your doctor to order a VAP cholesterol panel, thyroid function tests, vitamin D3, homocysteine, Lp(a), CPR, insulin, and a comprehensive blood chemistry panel.

These are the right tests and they could save your life.

Lifestyle

The *American College of Cardiology* 2004 national guidelines recommended therapeutic lifestyle changes as the standard of care in the management of cardiovascular disease (CVD) risk factors.[40] "Many patients with classic CVD risk factors can achieve risk-reduction goals without medication within three months of initiating therapeutic lifestyle changes".

The following highly respected organizations and others recommend therapeutic lifestyle changes as a first line therapy before prescribing pharmaceutical drugs for conditions most doctors see every day:

- National Institutes of Health[41]
- Center for Disease Control[42]
- American Heart Association[43]
- American Diabetes Association[44]

- North American Menopause Society[45]
- National Institute on Aging[46]

In our efforts to provide the best possible care both for patients with established CVD and those interested in CVD prevention, it is critical to recognize the positive impact of a healthy lifestyle. A combination of achieving ideal body weight, eating good, high-quality natural and organic foods and smaller portions, exercising at least two hours each week, having no addictions and regularly enjoying happiness—the best medicine in the world—will reduce your risk for all diseases by 70 percent, with no side effects. Making the right choices and seeking support to help guide you is a great investment in your life. You cannot put a price on your health.

The bottom line is to keep your cholesterol and your life in balance. Your life depends on it.

Chapter 10

TOXINS: RIGHT CHOICES

W e live in a toxic world. While making considerable technological advancements, we have generated environmental pollution with significant adverse health consequences worldwide. A frightening fact that you may not be aware of—the Environmental Protection Agency (EPA) has reported that 100 percent of human fat samples contain man-made chemicals.[1]

Toxic babies!

In 2004, the Environmental Working Group (EWG) tested 10 people for over 400 toxins. These 10 people had never been exposed to toxic air, contaminated water, pesticides in food or any environmental toxins. Their tests were positive for 287 chemicals. The test was done using the cord blood of newborn infants!

How shocking. We not only inherit genes but toxins as well. The blood of these newborns "harbored pesticides, a long list of consumer product ingredients, and waste from burning coal, gasoline, and garbage."

Among the toxins found were eight perfluorochemicals used as stain and oil repellants in fast food packaging, clothes and textiles—including the Teflon chemical PFOA, recently characterized as a likely human carcinogen by the EPA's Science Advisory Board. This chemical is found in dozens of widely used brominated flame retardants and their toxic by-products as well as numerous pesticides.

Of the 287 chemicals EWG detected in umbilical cord blood, we know that 180 cause cancers in humans or animals; 217 are toxic to the brain and nervous system, and 208 cause birth defects or abnormal development in animal tests. The dangers of pre- or post-natal exposure to this complex mixture of carcinogens, developmental toxins and neurotoxins have never been studied.

Children are at higher risks than adults when subjected to toxins:[2]

- A developing child's chemical exposures are greater pound-for-pound than those of adults.
- Children have lower levels of some chemical-binding proteins, allowing more of a chemical to reach "target organs."
- A baby's organs and systems are rapidly developing, and thus are often more vulnerable to damage from chemical exposure.
- Systems that detoxify and excrete industrial chemicals are not fully developed.
- The longer future life span of a child compared to an adult allows more time for adverse effects to arise.

Chemicals and toxins can be found in products we use every day. They are in your food, under the kitchen sink, in the basement and in the garage. They are in your body and on your face.

We have all heard the saying, "Beauty is only skin deep." But nothing could be further from the truth. Our skin is a reflection of our health. You have seen the radiant, beautiful skin of a healthy infant or a child. His eyes sparkle and her skin glows. You know the pale face of someone who is ill, the wrinkles and dry skin of someone who smokes or has a body filled with toxins and lacks proper nutrition. You have seen the face of someone who is stressed, tired or depressed.

Every half-inch square of skin contains 500,000 cells, 32 inches of blood vessels, 100 sweat glands, 21 inches of nerves, 15 oil glands and 230 sensory receptors. Your skin is very effective in absorbing whatever you put on it, including toxins!

Here's a surprise—anti-aging skin care products often contain toxins that over time damage and age the skin![3]

The average woman uses 12 products containing 168 different ingredients daily. Many cosmetic chemicals are designed to penetrate into the skin's inner layers, and they do. Consequently, some common cosmetic ingredients turn up in people's bodies. Among them are industrial plasticizers called phthalates, parabens, which are preservatives, and persistent fragrance components like musk xylene.

The beauty industry brags about the new technology to make skin care products using nanoparticles. Nanoparticles have received very little testing, yet because they are tiny particles they readily penetrate the skin and contaminate the body. Cosmetics manufacturers are not required to disclose the presence of nanoparticles in products. The Environmental Working Group (EWG) analysis has found that one-third of all personal care products on the market contain ingredients now commercially available in "nano" forms.[4]

The EWG is the creator of the Skin Deep Cosmetics Database.[5]

Are any levels of these chemicals found in our bodies causing biological damage? The risk is definite. Only more research will tell us the total damage after the fact.

Did you know that the Food and Drug Administration (FDA) have sponsored studies that have confirmed previous industry studies indicating that applying Alpha Hydroxy Acids (AHAs) to the skin results in increased UV sensitivity?[6] Products containing AHAs are made for a variety of purposes, such as smoothing fine lines, wrinkles, improving skin texture and tone, unblocking and cleansing pores, and improving the skin's condition in general.

The FDA has no authority to require cosmetic and personal care product companies to test products for safety. The FDA does not review or approve the vast majority of products or ingredients before they go on the market. The agency conducts pre-market reviews only for certain color additives and active ingredients in cosmetics classified as over-the-counter drugs.[7]

Even more shocking is that in its more than 30-year history, the industry's safety panel, the Cosmetic Ingredient Review (CIR), has assessed fewer than 20 percent of cosmetics ingredients and found only 11 ingredients or chemical groups to be unsafe, and its recommendations are not legally binding on companies. What this means is that over a 30-year period only 20 percent of the ingredients were ever tested, they were tested by the cosmetic industry itself.[8] This is certainly not an objective "research".

Of the estimated 85,000 chemicals in the U.S. marketplace, only a small fraction has ever been tested for chronic impacts to human health. While Europe has banned 1,100 chemicals from use in products, the U.S. has banned fewer than 10.

- More than 500 products sold in the U.S. contain ingredients banned in cosmetics in Japan, Canada or the European Union.[9]
- Nearly 100 products contain ingredients considered unsafe by the International Fragrance Association.[10]
- A wide range of nano materials whose safety is in question may be common in personal care products.[11]
- 22 percent of all personal care products may be contaminated with the cancer-causing impurity 1,4-dioxane, including many children's products.[12]
- 60 percent of sunscreens contain the potential hormone disruptor oxybenzone that readily penetrates the skin and contaminates the bodies of 97 percent of Americans.[13,14]
- 61 percent of tested lipstick brands contain residues of lead.[15]

When you see products labeled with "natural" or "organic", do your homework! Some of these often contain synthetic chemicals. Sometimes, even truly natural or organic ingredients are not necessarily risk-free. You need to do your research on every ingredient, since the cosmetics industry is virtually self-governing.

According to the BCC Research Group, "The global, plant-based pharmaceutical market, valued at $19.5 billion in 2008, relies on the ability of natural chemicals—like those used in some natural cosmetics—to significantly alter body functions, a far cry from innocuous."[16] On the other hand, products labeled "organic" or "natural" can contain petrochemicals and no certified organic or natural ingredients whatsoever. Products certified as organic can contain as little as 10 percent organic ingredients by weight or volume.[17]

The FDA tried establishing an official definition for the term "natural," but these protections were overturned in court.[18] Research shows that 35 percent of children's products marketed as "natural" contain artificial preservatives.[19]

It is astounding that the FDA has no authority to require recalls of harmful cosmetics. Furthermore, manufacturers are not required to report cosmetics-related injuries to the agency. The FDA relies on companies to report injuries voluntarily.[20]

One would think that regulations would already be in place to protect and inform consumers regarding products that contain cancer-causing chemicals and additives. The tobacco industry has a warning label on their packaging—there needs to be some consistency. We have a right to know in order to make an informed decision.

"Research has shown that many conventional personal-care products contain chemicals of concern that can disrupt your hormones, have been linked to cancer, cause allergies or can damage your skin," explains Stacy Malkan, author of *Not Just a Pretty Face: The Ugly Side of the Beauty Industry.*[21] She heads up the advocacy group, the Campaign for Safe Cosmetics, and maintains an online list of chemicals she says are dangerous. She points out that because the U.S. has few safety standards for cosmetics, "companies are basically making their own decisions about what's safe enough to sell."

A few common skin-care toxins to avoid are:

- Sodium lauryl or laureth sulfate
- Petroleum, paraffin, and mineral oil
- Parabens
- Propylene glycol and phthalates

- Toluene
- Aluminum
- Lead
- Dioxane

Sodium Lauryl Sulfate

What do cleansers, shampoos, bubble bath and toothpaste have in common with garage floor cleaners and engine degreasers? Sodium Lauryl Sulfate (SLS).

Sodium lauryl or laureth sulfate is used in more than 90 percent of our personal skin care products. Sodium laurel breaks down the skin's moisture barriers and easily penetrates the skin. It can also cause hair loss. It is in a class called *nitrosamines*, a potent class of carcinogens. SLS is reported to be the most frequent cause of eye irritation by shampoos. SLS can damage the protective outer layer of the skin, and has been shown through research to penetrate the skin to a depth of 1/4 inch, causing skin irritation—with deeper penetration occurring throughout the body.

Using cosmetics and personal hygiene products containing SLS can allow other toxicants to penetrate the skin more easily. Health experts at The National Institute of Health (NIH) state the health risks from skin care products pose a greater risk to public health than smoking.

Only 17 percent of sunscreens are both safe and effective. The incidence of skin cancer and melanomas has not decreased since the use of sunscreen over the last 25 years. The facts are that several studies in the 1990s reported a higher, not lower, incidence of a very deadly skin cancer, malignant melanoma in which sunscreen was used frequently.[22,23,24,25]

- Squamous cell skin cancer may decrease with the use of sunscreen.
- Basal cell carcinomas have not decreased with sunscreen use.

Parabens

Parabens are a group of widely used preservatives added to food and cosmetics, and an extremely common ingredient in underarm deodorants and antiperspirants. These chemicals have come under scrutiny in recent years because in studies on animals and cells they have demonstrated an estrogenic (hormonal) effect; therefore you should avoid deodorants and antiperspirants containing parabens and aluminum.

A Danish study of 26 healthy male volunteers who applied cosmetic creams containing parabens detected the substances in their bloodstreams within one hour. Dr. Philippa Darbre, an oncologist, performed a study which showed that parabens could be detected in human breast tissue.[26]

Personal care products, especially deodorants and antiperspirants containing parabens, have been linked to breast cancer since they are applied close to the breast where they could potentially adhere to DNA and encourage the development of damaged cells.

Aluminum Salts

Another cause for concern in underarm products is aluminum salts, which are authorized to be used at high levels in antiperspirants, sometimes making up to 25 percent of the product. A recent report from the Department of Biomolecular Sciences in Italy found that fluid taken from the nipples of cancer patients contained nearly twice the aluminum compared with nipple fluid taken from women without breast cancer.[27] Large amounts of aluminum salts can also be found in many vaccines such as hepatitis and tetanus. Studies have also shown that over time, this aluminum is slowly dispersed throughout the entire body.

Lead

Lead is a neurotoxin in popular black hair dyes for men and women. Lead from hair dyes travels from hair to doorknobs, cabinets and other household items, where children have access to it, making hair dye extremely toxic in any environment.

Several of my patients who were tested by a specific lab proved to have diaminobenzene stuck to their DNA. Some of these patients presented with neurological disorders and others with chronic illness. Diaminobenzene is found in hair dyes and shampoos.

Fortunately, specific intravenous (IV) lipid based protocols can be effective in removing toxins. Using these IV protocols, the toxins were removed from their DNA, which was confirmed in the repeat lab test. The bottom line is that the damage that toxins create to our health is not pretty.

The FDA's new study found lead in 400 lipsticks tested (primarily red shades), with higher lead levels than ever reported in some of the most popular brands. The worst offender was L'Oreal USA, who's Maybelline Color Sensation and L'Oreal Color Riche lipsticks were number one and number two on the list. In fact, L'Oreal USA makes five of the 10 most contaminated brands in the FDA study.[28]

A brand new report for the U.S. Centers for Disease Control (CDC) states there is no safe level of lead exposure for children.[29] This means we must protect women from lead exposure, since lead builds up in the body over time and easily crosses the placenta where it can interfere with normal development of a fetus and cause irreversible negative health effects. Beauty industry officials contend that the risks of using cosmetics with trace amounts of chemicals are insignificant or nonexistent.

Formaldehyde

Formaldehyde is a suspected carcinogen and common skin and eye irritant. The International Agency for Research on Cancer says there is evidence formaldehyde causes a form of throat cancer in humans.[30] The FDA does not object to the use of formaldehyde in cosmetics.

Formaldehyde is used as a preservative in nail polishes, soaps, Brazilian Blowout and other cosmetic products. It is also found in household products such as furniture polish.

In November 2011, an advocacy group found that Johnson & Johnson was selling baby shampoo in the United States, Canada and several other countries containing small amounts of quaternium-15, a formaldehyde-releasing preservative that has been linked to cancer, even though the company had removed the chemical from similar products sold in Europe and Japan.[31]

The company has announced it did not believe the small amounts in its shampoos posed any threat but it would phase out the use of such ingredients across the globe. To Johnson and Johnson's credit they have recently said they will remove toxins from their products.[32]

A potent preservative considered to be a known human carcinogen by the International Agency on Research on Cancer, formaldehyde, also is an asthmagen, neurotoxicant and developmental toxicant, and was once mixed into many personal care products as an antiseptic agent. This use has declined. But some hair straighteners are based on formaldehyde's hair-stiffening action and release substantial amounts of the chemical, especially when exposed to heat. Many common preservatives also release formaldehyde into products (like DMDM hydantoin, quaternium, and urea compounds).[33]

Other Products containing harmful toxins:

Dandruff Shampoos:

Most of the active ingredients approved by the FDA for use in dandruff shampoos have significant safety concerns. Common dandruff control ingredients—selenium sulfide, ketoconazole, salicylic acid, and coal tar—are identified on the European or California list of carcinogens and/or reproductive toxicants.[34] They can also cause minor to significant skin reactions, including irritation, inflammation and photosensitivity. These products should be used sparingly and only as directed. Avoid using dandruff shampoo on children, especially to treat benign conditions like cradle cap and normal scalp flaking.

The concern isn't just one chemical in your or your child's shampoo, but rather the buildup of potentially dangerous additives from a variety of sources. "The toxic exposures just add up over time," says Barbara Sattler, director of the Environmental Health Education Center at the University Of Maryland School Of Nursing. "If you've got a set of neurotoxins in two or three or five products you're using and you're putting them on your skin and inhaling or ingesting them every day, you're increasing the risk of an untoward effect," she explains in a recent *Washington Post* article.

Antibacterial products (soaps, antiperspirants, toothpaste):

Triclosan is one of the most common over the counter (OTC) antibacterial chemicals found in personal care products such as antibacterial soaps. However, triclosan-based soaps are not any more effective than plain soap and water.

Triclosan is also very toxic to the environment and may disrupt hormonal function in people and other mammals.[35]

The issue is the lifelong accumulation of toxins that raises serious health concerns. As these accumulate day after day, week after week, month after month and year after year, what is the biological damage? And what is the environmental damage as well? Only the research will tell *after the fact*. The fact is, because individuals vary their ability to detoxify the severity of damage is personal.

One thing is for sure. It is not good!

As a result, it's your choice whether to use a fruity body wash, lipstick or after-shave which may contain lead, diethyl phthalate (a hormone disruptor widely used in plastics and linked to sperm damage and other reproductive problems) or 1,4-Dioxane, a carcinogenic byproduct that has been banned in Europe, which has also been deemed as a cancer-causing agent here in the U.S.[36]

The green sector of the cosmetics industry is booming, and those who want to avoid toxins have a wealth of options. However, experts say caution is warranted. "Unfortunately, there's a lot of 'green washing' that goes on: pretending that a product is green when it's really not," says Stacy Malkan, "and since it's not regulated, relying on marketing claims or labels isn't your best bet." You can read for yourself and then decide what products to keep from your bathroom cabinet.

Furthermore, 'hypoallergenic' and 'dermatologist tested' are two frequently used terms. Since they are not legal terms and they can be put on any label such as on a can of gasoline. They unfortunately may bear little or no relation to the product inside.

Always check your personal care and beauty products before you make your purchase. Check out the EWG website for the least toxic skin care products.

Plastics and Their Evils

Plastic is everywhere. It's used in consumer products and packaging of all kinds. And while it solves a lot of problems for manufacturers and can seem convenient to consumers, its widespread use causes serious risk to human health and the environment. Three plastics have been shown to leach toxic chemicals when heated, worn, or put under pressure:

- Polycarbonate, which leaches Bisphenol A (BPA).
- PVC, or polyvinyl chloride, which leaches phthalates.
- Polystyrene, which leaches styrene.

BPA is one of the most pervasive chemicals in modern life. It's a building block of polycarbonate plastic (often labeled recycle #7) and is used in thousands of consumer products, including food packaging. Research shows BPA exposure is linked to breast cancer.[37]

The more plastics we have in our bodies, the higher the risk for disease. "Higher BPA (Bisphenol A, a plastic) exposure may be associated with avoidable mortality. There is a strong relationship between Bisphenol A and the risk of CVD, type 2 diabetes, and liver enzyme abnormalities," reported the *Journal of the American Medical Association* in 2008.[38]

When our bodies contain toxins like plastics, the liver produces an enzyme called Gamma-glutamyltransferase (GGT) in an effort to make glutathione, a powerful antioxidant that can neutralize toxins. GGT is associated with an increased risk of CVD, diabetes, high cholesterol, high C-reactive protein and toxins. Elevated GGT is also found in patients with Parkinson's disease.

Phthalates are a group of endocrine-disrupting chemicals found in PVC (#3 plastic). Phthalate exposure has been linked to early puberty in girls, a risk factor for later-life breast cancer. Some phthalates also act as weak estrogens in cell culture systems. A growing number of studies also link this chemical to male reproductive system disorders. Everyone should avoid products with "fragrance" indicating a chemical mixture that may contain phthalates.

Vinyl chloride and dioxin, which are endocrine disruptors, are formed in the manufacturing of polyvinyl chloride (PVC) (#3 plastic). These are two of the first chemicals designated as known human carcinogens by the National Toxicology Program and the International Agency for Research on Cancer. They have also been linked to increased mortality from breast cancer among workers involved in their manufacturing.[39]

Are you drinking a carcinogen as you enjoy your coffee latte? **Styrene** can leach from polystyrene or #6 plastic and is found in Styrofoam food trays, egg cartons, disposable cups and bowls, carryout containers and opaque plastic cutlery. It has been classified by the International Agency for Research on Cancer as a human carcinogen.[40]

Many of these chemicals as well as others such as lead, mercury, PCBs, pesticides and solvents are known to be harmful to a child's developing brain. They can contribute to learning, behavioral and developmental disabilities.

According to the National Environmental Trust Physicians for Social Responsibility Learning Disabilities Association of America, "The U.S. Census Bureau estimates that 12 million U.S. children (17 percent of all children) suffer from one or more developmental, learning, or behavioral disabilities. The National Academy of Sciences recently estimated that about three percent of developmental and neurological defects in children are caused by exposure to known toxic substances—including drugs, cigarette smoke, and known developmental and neurological toxins like lead, PCBs, and mercury.

"This means that 360,000 U.S. children (1 in every 200 U.S. children) suffer from developmental or neurological deficits caused by exposure to known toxic substances. In fact, one out of every six children in the U.S. has a neurological disorder and researchers are finding evidence linking this disability to common household chemicals."[41]

Mercury is especially toxic. The FDA recommends that people eat albacore tuna once a week at most and chunk tuna no more than twice a week. Pregnant women (or those trying to conceive) should avoid high-mercury fish as much as possible.[42] What is striking to me is that dentists are still putting mercury on children's and adult's teeth and worse yet—they are removing amalgam without the safety precautions. Look for Board Certified Biological Dentists—they know how to remove these toxic amalgams safely.

Avoiding toxins as much as possible is the best way to keep healthy; don't store food in plastic, don't put plastic in the dishwasher and don't heat food in plastic in the microwave, unless of course, you are craving plastics and enjoy eating them.

Pesticides in our Food

Each year nearly a billion pounds of pesticides are sprayed in fields and orchards across the country, contaminating our food. Think of it this way. Pesticides need to be toxic to kill pests. If the bugs won't eat it we shouldn't either.

Infants and children are especially vulnerable to pesticides. Playing in the grass, on the floor or putting objects in their mouth increases the risk for toxin exposure. Their bodies are small and not fully developed so they are not efficient in removing toxins. The consumption of food and water is greater per body weight in smaller children than in adults which increases their risk for pesticides and toxins.[43]

What are the most toxic fruits? In a study, 98 percent of conventional apples were found to contain pesticides. Celery is highly contaminated and tested positive for 57 different pesticides. Strawberries, a delicious snack, expose us to as many as 13 different pesticides. Due to the constant use of pesticides, many other foods are contaminated.[44] The Dirty Dozen (most highly saturated produce with pesticides listed in order of worst contamination to least): apples, celery, sweet bell peppers, peaches, strawberries, imported nectarines, grapes, spinach, lettuce, cucumbers, domestic blueberries, potatoes.[45]

Go to EWG.org and get the list of The Dirty Dozen.

The USDA's Nationwide Food Consumption Surveys[46] provides information on what people eat or what is a "typical meal." Total Diet Studies are designed to determine pesticide residues in commonly eaten menu items such as macaroni and cheese, chicken nuggets, popcorn and ice cream.

The three most common residues found in such studies were the insecticides DDT, malathion and chlorpyrifos-methyl. These residues were not above the acceptable or tolerance limits.[46] It really is unbelievable and alarming to know that there are so called "acceptable or tolerance limits" on DDT, malathion and chloprpyrifos-methyl.

Even worse, not everything in a product can be found on the label. Right now, there's absolutely no requirement to label foods that have been genetically engineered (with genetically modified organisms—GMOs). EWG has already asked the FDA to require labeling of genetically-engineered ingredients in the food we eat.[47]

Extensive research shows that it is not a question of **if** we are carrying a burden of these toxins, but rather how much and to what extent they affect our health. Exposure to toxins such as chemicals, heavy metals (lead, cadmium, mercury) and "bugs" such as parasites, viruses, bacteria and fungi have become part of our world that are hard to avoid and challenging to remove from our tissues. These toxins can affect every part of our body, including our brain and sex organs.

Consider this; according to the U.S. Environmental Protection Agency[48] in 2010…

- 20,904 facilities reported to Toxics Release Inventory (TRI). Together they reported total on- and off-site disposal or other releases of 3.93 billion pounds of toxic chemicals. Most were disposed of or released on-site to land, air or water, or injected underground.[48]
- Over 0.23 billion pounds of chemicals were discharged into surface waters (i.e., lakes, rivers and oceans).[48]
- Nearly 0.86 billion pounds of air emissions were pumped into the atmosphere.[48]
- We ingest more than 30 to 50 tons of food in a lifetime. Like air and water, most food is laden with numerous chemicals that need to be detoxified properly—otherwise they are deposited in various tissues.
- Several thousand food additives are intentionally added to our food supply and thousands more slip into our food supply unintentionally during harvesting, processing or packaging. In fact, the average American consumes about 124 pounds of food additives a year![49]
- More than 400 pesticides and herbicides are currently licensed for use on food and crops.[50]

The two most important things we need to know to create health and cure disease are:

The Role of Toxins and the Importance of Detoxification

The poor nutritional value of our food is further complicated by the extraordinary amounts of toxic chemicals in our food and in our bodies. As our external environment has radically changed, so has the internal environment of our bodies.

The good news is that specialty lab tests can determine if you have plastics, pesticides, heavy metals, PCBs, or volatile solvents in your body. They can be removed using specific supplements or intravenous therapies.

Detoxification

Detoxification is the process of the elimination of toxic "sludge" we are carrying inside our bodies. This sludge, as I prefer to call it, also decreases our libido. That is just one of the many important reasons to remove it.

Do you have fatigue, muscle aches, headaches, concentration and memory problems, fibromyalgia, chemical sensitivities, negative reactions to certain foods, sensitivity to medications or a family history of a neurological disorder? If so, your body may be toxic and crying out for help. To approach illness and disease, one must begin with the health of the cell membrane.

If you have an elevated GGT, exposures to toxins or a neurological disorder, you may benefit from an intravenous infusion of glutathione.

The tri-peptide glutathione acts as an immune system booster and a detoxifier. Glutathione is produced by the liver. Often called "the master antioxidant," glutathione is required by all other antioxidants—even vitamins C and E—to function properly. Also described as "food for the immune system," glutathione is not well-absorbed orally; however it can be given in higher doses intravenously and will go directly to the cells via the blood system.

Also, supplementing with EPH/DHA, evening primrose oil, PC, short chain fatty acid butyrate, vitamin D3 and supplements can also help your body detoxify.

Thankfully, the human body has an extraordinary capacity for resiliency, regeneration, repair, recovery and renewal. Detoxification is about resting, cleansing, and nourishing the body from the inside out. The effectiveness of detoxification is dependent on the cell's membrane and the structure of specific lipids (fats).

Patients, like many others suffering from toxicity, often experience tremendous discomfort, confusion and pain in their state of illness. Healing the body and brain requires precise nourishment and targeted detoxification to release the burden of toxicity. Taking good care of oneself is an important part of the healing process, especially when in a state of toxicity.

While there are numerous ways to detoxify and new detoxification programs added daily, the basic principles remain the same and must always involve detoxification on a cellular level to be effective, restore health and have long-lasting results. To be effective, detoxification must include the cell membrane.

When the cell membrane is healthy, fluid and active in the detoxification process, the decrease of symptoms and the restoration back to health is dramatic. Of the tens of thousands of molecules that make up the life of a cell, phosphatidylcholine (PC) stands apart; it is the most important part of the cell membrane.

The membrane is the structural skin that surrounds the cell. It is far more than an outside layer—it is literally the essence of life. You may damage other parts of the cell, even the nucleus and the DNA, and the cell will still carry on. But damage the membrane and the cell is gone.

This membrane is the lining of every nerve cell that carries our signals. It manages the production of energy. It manages all of our senses. The sheer volume of the membrane in the body is mind-bending. The liver alone has about 300,000 square feet of membrane. That's more than 4 football fields—4.63 to be exact.

Basically, detoxification means cleaning the blood. The proper form of detoxification occurs on a cellular level. It does this mainly by removing impurities from the blood in the liver, where toxins are processed for elimination. The body also eliminates toxins through the kidneys, intestines, lungs, lymph and skin. However, when this system is compromised and impurities aren't properly filtered through the cell wall, then every cell in the body is adversely affected and the organs cannot detoxify.

Dr. Patricia Kane, PhD, has developed an international reputation for her expertise in detoxification, essential fatty acids and their effect on membrane function. The translation of tens of thousands of papers and through her clinical experience with thousands of patients, Dr. Kane has created an innovative and clinically effective series of interventions. Her research and work has helped many patients using lipid based IV protocols as a therapy for effective detoxification and healing.

Her life's work has been computerized, allowing an individual's biomarkers to be fed into a huge database of over 30,000 research papers and in the blink of an eye, the exact nutrients they may need to improve their health can be identified.

The work of K. J. Gundermann, PhD, MD, is also noteworthy in his book, *The Essential Phospholipids as a Membrane Therapeutic.*[51] It covers extensively the use of PC in toxicity, hematology, alcohol and diabetic fatty liver, lung, psoriasis, elevated lipids and atherosclerosis.

The PK protocol, based on more than 20 years of research, is an intravenous administration of PC, folinic acid (the bioavailable form of folic acid) and glutathione. Glutathione strongly aids liver detoxification. Vitamin C and selenium support glutathione production. Each protocol can be customized to the individual based on their medical history, symptoms and data from the lab analysis.

Genes + Environment = Disease

Some of us are better detoxifiers than others. Individuals may have genetic detoxification impairments. These are called Single Nucleotide Polymorphisms, or SNPs which can be determined by a lab test. This is important as it gives specific information regarding what medications and toxins are important to avoid because of a specific gene variation. We know that many things affect how our genes work—our diet, vitamins and minerals, toxins, allergens, infections, stress, lack of sleep, exercise and more.

About 20 percent of the population carries the Apo E4 gene which may affect mercury detoxification. Having an inefficient GST gene can result in lower levels of glutathione, the body's main detoxifier and antioxidant. A DNA test, MTHFR, can determine the body's ability to methylate, an important part of detoxification.

We also know genes are not our destiny. They are like light switches. You can boost your ability by turning on the right genes and turning off the wrong ones.

Detoxification Steps to Lighten Up Your Toxin Load:

- Eliminate alcohol, coffee, cigarettes, refined sugars and saturated fats, all of which act as toxins in the body and are obstacles to your healing process.
- Eat organic
- Avoid artificially-colored foods
- Avoid snacks loaded with hydrogenated oils, sugar, salt, and corn syrup
- Do not eat processed meats such as hot dogs, bacon, and sausage as they contain nitrosamines which are carcinogenic.
- Eat small fish and avoid large ones loaded with mercury. Fish from the deep, cold North Atlantic and Norwegian waters are the purest.
- Skip the artificial sweeteners containing aspartame, a nervous system toxin.
- Minimize use of chemical-based household cleaners and personal health care products (cleansers, shampoos, deodorants and toothpastes) and substitute natural alternatives.
- Eat plenty of fiber, including brown rice and organically grown fresh fruits and vegetables. Beets, radishes, artichokes, cabbage, broccoli, spirulina, chlorella and seaweed are excellent detoxifying foods.
- Take vitamins, essential fatty acids, minerals and amino acids as needed.
- Drink at least eight glasses of water daily.
- Breathe deeply to allow oxygen to circulate more completely through your system.
- Exercise.
- Eat less.
- Transform stress by emphasizing positive emotions.
- Use a sauna so your body can eliminate wastes through perspiration.
- Use specific intravenous protocol individualized for you for faster and more effective detoxification.

Remember, life is on the cell membrane. Nourishing our cells heals the body and heals the brain.

The Critical Role of Nutrition

The average person eats 29 pounds of French fries, 23 pounds of pizza, 24 pounds of ice cream and consumes 53 gallons of soda, 24 pounds of artificial sweeteners, 2.736 pounds of salt and 90,700 milligrams of caffeine per year.[52] Do we really think we can create health in such a toxic environment? Do we really think we can have beautiful skin and hair while eating processed food, saturated fat and preservatives?

Many women experience hair loss. A normal cycle of hair growth is two to three years, growing about a half inch per month. Ninety percent of hair is growing while 10 percent is resting. After about two to three months, the resting hair falls out. Approximately 30 million women have noticeable hair loss.[53] Hair loss may be due to illness, medications, and/or hormones. Hidden food allergies and gluten sensitivity are common root causes of hair loss. For healthy hair and skin good nutrition is essential.

- Vitamin A helps to secret sebum.
- Vitamin E increases circulation.
- Vitamin B keeps hairs firm on the scalp.

If you have crackling, scaling skin you may be deficient in vitamin B3 (niacin). In addition to skin and hair, B3 is important for energy, digestion, the nervous system, and the eyes and mouth. It helps to eliminate toxins and support the production of sex hormones. B3 is found in beets, brewer's yeast, meat, poultry, fish, seeds and nuts.

Vitamin B6, biotin, folate, and pantothenate are good for your skin. Sixty percent of individuals have a genetic modification which impairs their ability to convert folic acid into folate, which helps the body detoxify heavy metals and other toxins. Therefore, folate should be methylated (a methyl group should be added) to help our bodies use it properly.

Do you have dry skin and hair, eczema or psoriasis? It's important to eat an adequate amount of omega 3 and omega 6 essential fatty acids as excellent quality fish oil, organic cold pressed sunflower oil, safflower oil, hemp see oil (Canadian source), phosphatidylcholine, raw nuts and seeds for your brain, body and beauty.

If you are healthy and eating well but still experiencing hair loss, it could be due to low stomach acid. According to Gaby, Alan MD, *Nutritional Medicine*, 2011. 50 percent of people 50 years or older and 85 percent of people over the age of 80 have low stomach acid. Obviously, 100 percent of individuals on antacids have low stomach acid.

Stomach acid is important for two reasons: one, to digest your food, and two, to kill off the bacteria, viruses and parasites we eat on a daily basis. According to the *Journal of the American Medical Association*, if you have low stomach acid, not only will nutrient deficiencies cause more problems with your skin and hair, but all the organs in your body will be affected.[54]

Food Allergies and Your Skin

The skin is a great detoxifier. We are familiar with signs such as a rash from a virus or a bacterial infection, or hives from a food allergy. Skin conditions are a sign something else in the body is out of balance, sick or toxic.

Do you or your teenager suffer from acne? Acne is a common condition characterized by papules or pustules. Possible causes can be infection, tissue inflammation, plugged hair follicles, nutrient deficiencies and/or hormonal imbalances. Nutrient deficiencies include zinc, vitamin A, vitamin B6, vitamin C and selenium.

According to Dr. Alan Gaby in *Nutritional Medicine*, 2011, numerous investigators have reported that a hidden allergy or sensitivity to foods is a major contributing factor in some cases of acne.[55]

Exacerbations of acne can result from allergic reactions or from the effects of biologically active substances in certain foods (e.g., hormones in cow's milk and possibly amines or other chemicals in chocolate). In one study, restricting sugar in soft drinks, fruit drinks, candy and cake resulted in an 84 percent substantial improvement or complete clearing of acne lesions. Like most signs and symptoms, skin conditions may have a combination of causes.

Food allergies can be easily detected in a lab by testing 90 different foods. The results can change your life by decreasing inflammation to improve your health and your beauty!

GI Effects

If you are suffering from IBS or are even not experiencing any symptoms, you may have a hidden infection, causing decreased digestion or absorption of foods. If you have any signs of inflammation the underlying cause could be a problem your intestines. This can have a huge impact on your skin, hair, teeth and overall health. A specific gastrointestinal tract test that checks the DNA often is the key to restoring your health. You cannot afford to miss this diagnosis.

Will Rogers said, "Some people try to turn back their odometers. Not me—I want people to know why I look this way. I have traveled a long way and some of the roads weren't paved." Most people other than Will Rogers want fewer wrinkles. Wrinkles and photo-aging may result from age, sun, smoking, nutrient deficiencies, low stomach acid or toxic skin care products.

Check the labels on your skin and hair products. Do not put anything on your skin you would not eat, because it is all absorbed into your blood stream. This means if it would not be safe to eat your toothpaste, shampoo or hair dye, then don't use it.

Many sources are available for safer and less toxic skin care products.

See www.safecosmetics.org or www.whitelotusliving.com.

Products made by compounding pharmacies are effective so you can be both safe and beautiful, but always read your labels.

The best thing to do is to clean up!

- Be tested to find out what toxins may be lurking in your body.
- Have as many toxins as possible removed from your body.
- Choose a Board Certified Biological Dentist.
- Become much more attuned to clean living—eat organic foods; use personal skin care products and sunscreens deemed safe; drink only filtered water.
- Read labels carefully.
- Wash foods well, but not with soap!
- Peel fruits and vegetables after washing.

• Search the websites www.ewg.org and www.womenandenvironment. org for information on the safest cosmetics, sunscreen, drinking water, food, and household products.

Beauty is more than skin deep! Laughter, clean living and natural products will make you healthier and happier—and that's what beauty is all about!

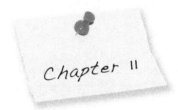

Chapter 11

THE FORK IN THE ROAD: GETTING IT RIGHT

The question is "Is the life you are living worth the life you are giving up?" What is your answer?

Things didn't used to be so difficult. You may be just trying to make it through the day. You are smiling for your family and the public, but the smile isn't real. You are not well but you don't want to complain. Gone are the days that you had left over energy at the end of day. The days when you could multitask. The days you experienced boundless enthusiasm. You notice you need two of everything…2 pair of glasses, 2 pair of sunglasses, 2 sets of keys just in case you can't find the first item.

I want you to know you are not alone. Don't give up. There is help and there is hope.

Janet came into my office after seeing many physicians over several years. She said she was exhausted, and as she said it she had tears in her eyes. She said in a desperate tone, "You are my last hope." Janet was unable to work and spent much of her day in bed with pain. Her symptoms also included migraines, sinusitis, anxiety, depression, heartburn, irritable bowel disease, joint pain, muscle stiffness, difficulty concentrating, lack of focus, and memory loss. Her extensive medical records revealed a normal chemistry panel, negative endoscopy and colonoscopy. The diagnoses were "normal findings" and the recommendations from her previous doctor were an antacid and an SSRI anti-depressant.

After a comprehensive assessment and specialized lab tests, Janet was found to have severe IgG hidden food allergies, low thyroid, and a neurotransmitter imbalance. A DNA stool test also diagnosed intestinal parasites, H. Pylori, and intestinal overgrowth of yeast. She was treated for these conditions using natural therapies whenever possible. She discontinued her antacid and antidepressant. After 3 months, all of her symptoms disappeared and she was happy, healthy, productive, and back to work full time!

In Janet's own words.

> *"Dr. Norling changed my life. I was just existing, performing minimal duties with absolutely no passion, lacking motivation and energy. My self-esteem was minimal, I had severe indigestion and would become full after a few bites of food. Dr. Norling's diagnosis was food allergies (dairy and eggs), extreme Vitamin D deficiency and H-Pylori bacteria. She also tested my neurotransmitters and found that I had low levels of gaba, serotonin and dopamine. I was given supplements and I have never felt better in my life. She explained that we have as many brain cells (neurons) in our gut as our brain, so the food allergies were causing brain fog. I wake up every day excited about my life. Dr. Norling has also treated my four year old grandson, I believe saving his life. In addition she has treated my six year old grandson's food allergies and gut issues, and six other members of my family, the rest are waiting in line. We are indebted to Dr. Norling and her treatment of the body, mind and spirit."*

The landscape of healthcare and clinical practice are changing quickly, with more and more people today developing chronic illness, chronic pain, and unresolving conditions. Many of these individuals do not have a "diagnosable disease".

They have a long list of symptoms and ailments but using the conventional testing today, they are dismissed, overlooked, and misdiagnosed by a hurried doctor. The conventional labs are normal and you look good on paper. But you know you are not well. You know you just don't have the energy, stamina, and mental clarity you once enjoyed.

Dr. Jeffrey Bland says, "We need to listen to the patients' story and develop a response to it. The approach to complex syndromes may be much more profound than just trying to point a round peg in a square hole and get a singular diagnosis."

Natural Approach to Total Fitness

Busy lives, stressful schedules, poor diets, inadequate sleep, not enough down time and lack of energy are all too common in our society today. With all of life's obligations, something has got to give, and often it's your fitness regimen.

It's time for a change. It can be challenging to find time to work out, but the long and short-term health benefits make it a necessary aspect of achieving optimum health. Everyone has time to start exercising at least 15 minutes a day. It may help to view exercise and fitness as tools not just for the physical body. They are for the mind, body, and spirit as well.

Mental Fitness

Scientific studies studies show there is a close connection between our mind, body, thoughts, and emotions. When you have a joyful thought or feel gratitude, your brain releases a cascade of molecules and feel good hormones that elevate your mood and strengthen your immune system.

On the other hand, when you stuck in a negative emotional turbulence and painful thoughts caused by past experiences or injury or illness, you are likely to experience the physical symptoms of stress and disease, such a fatigue, chronic pain, and digestive issues.

Let it go. You deserve better than hauling all that old destructive baggage with you.

Just as physical exercise maintains body tone, strength, and endurance, mental exercise has positive conditioning affects as well. The National Institute of Mental Health, Duke University, and the National Institute on Aging support the findings that "mental and physical decline with aging is not inevitable."

Today I see more and more patients, ages 30 and older, who complain about short-term memory loss, difficulty focusing and concentrating and sluggish thinking. We need to re-energize and exercise our brain.

Eating six, small, well-balanced meals a day helps to maintain blood sugar levels and enables us to think clearly. Relief of stress, balanced biochemistry, and healthy lifestyle changes promoting optimal health are foundations for mental fitness.

The first step is to take action! Overcome monotony and routine in your life as it generates mental and emotional lethargy and resignation. Our brains are wired to be curious, but sometimes our busy lives stifle or deny us of our natural curiosity.

- Laugh—Laughing helps reduce stress and breaks old patterns. It can be a "quick-charge" for our brains.
- Remember—Spend time with your positive memories.
- Play—Take time to play. It is a great way to exercise your brain.
- Learn something new—Whatever you decide to learn can be light, fun, and distracting. Exercise your brain by learning and enjoy the increase of endorphins!
- Exercise—Physical activity brings more oxygen to the brain.
- Feed your brain—Essential fatty acids, EPA/DHA, good nutrition and supporting supplements will provide you with a clear mind.
- Rest more—Your brain works well with adequate rest and sleep.

Schedule these activities on your smart phone. Your brain will thank you in the form of new ideas, greater stamina, and more passion for your life.

Emotional Fitness

Stress can be thought of as a message from our central nervous system. It's telling us that enough is most definitely enough, and if we don't provide some relief, it is going to take other systems down with it! Physical exercise is good for developing a lean body, strong muscles and a strong heart, but is has also been shown to help maintain emotional fitness as well! In fact, researchers at Duke University studied people suffering from depression for four months and found that 60 percent of the participants who exercised for 30 minutes just three times a week overcame their depression without using antidepressant medication.[1]

Even more surprising, one study found that workouts as short as eight minutes in length could help alleviate feelings of sadness, tension and anger, along with improving resistance to disease in healthy people. Keep in mind that exercise also boosts confidence and reduces anxiety and stress, all of which contribute to psychological health and well-being. For example, Yoga participants often say they feel more centered and calm in addition to the physical benefits of stretching and building strength.

Emotional fitness starts by remembering what is important. Most of what stresses us are things that don't matter in the long run. Being cut off in traffic, breaking a fingernail, not being able to buy the newest gadget and someone else's rudeness are just not worth worrying about. Our family, our friends, and our health are what really matter.

Daniel Goleman, author of the best-seller, *Emotional Intelligence* and his more recent book, *Working with Emotional Intelligence*, emphasizes that the stronger we are in our self-awareness, self-regulation, motivation, empathy and social skills, the more successful and healthy we are likely to be. That said; keep these tips in mind when maintaining emotional wellness:

- Nurture your relationships—Spend quality time with the people you love. It doesn't matter how busy you are.
- Ask for help—It isn't in the nature of a lot of people to *ask* for help, but you'll be amazed when you do.
- Cry—Go ahead, get it over with. You'll feel better.

- Accept and Embrace—it is okay that you can't do everything and that you aren't perfect.
- Breathe—Take deep, calming breaths often.
- Take a nice long bath—Add one cup of Epsom salts or sea salt. You'll feel like you're in Heaven.
- Go to the spa for a weekend—This isn't pampering. This is good health.

Physical Fitness

In the past two decades, the proportion of children and teens in America who are overweight or obese has tripled. Nine million kids are carrying excess weight, with millions more at serious risk. Television and computer games have taken the place of physical activity for many American children; with more kids playing football on their PlayStation than they are on the playground.

If the trend continues, this generation of school children may be the first in modern times to have a *shorter* life expectancy than their parents. According to the *Journal of the American Medical Association*, an eight-year study of 13,000 people found that those who walked 30 minutes a day had a significantly lower risk of premature death than those who rarely exercised. In fact, a regular walking program can help reduce blood cholesterol, lower blood pressure, increase cardiovascular endurance, boost bone strength, burn calories, and keep weight down. Best of all, walking is simple, free, and convenient. If you are just beginning a fitness plan, walking is a great place to start:

- Walk short distances—Begin with a five-minute stroll and gradually increase your distance.
- Forget about speed—Walk at a comfortable pace. Focus on good posture, keeping your head lifted and shoulders relaxed.
- Swing your arms naturally—Breathe deeply. If you can't catch your breath, slow down or avoid hills.
- Be sure you can talk while walking—If you can't talk, you are walking too fast.

Everyone can use help getting fit. Work with professionals who can support your path to health and fitness. All you have to do is begin, keep trying, and remember that small steps bring big rewards.

Are your Mind, Body, and Spirit fit?

Mental Fitness

- You feel alert most of the time.
- You read or study regularly.
- You engage regularly in mental exercises.
- You are stimulated by new problems.
- You play and you rest.

Emotional Fitness

- You feel good about your life.
- You feel confident about your abilities and are aware of your weaknesses.
- You feel comfortable whether alone or in the presence of other people.
- You can handle change and challenges with a positive attitude.
- When you feel frustrated, you believe you can change things for the better.
- You remember what is important.

Physical Fitness

- Your weight is within the suggested healthy limits for your height, sex and age.
- Your body feels good.
- You exercise regularly.
- You have an annual physical exam and appropriate diagnostic tests regularly.
- You eat lots of vegetables and fruit, drink plenty of water and avoid trans fats (margarine) and those high in sugar.
- You have stamina and flexibility.

Spiritual Fitness
- You have a sense of meaning and purpose in your life.
- You take time to be in nature and take notice of it.
- You spend time developing your creative side.
- You feel connected with the world.
- You love the mystery of life!

In general, to live a healthy life:
- Find the underlying cause of your illness.
- Test the levels of the nutrients in your body.
- Use the best supplements and IV therapies.
- Add love and laughter to your life.

Enhance Your Lifestyle... Enhance Your Life

Would you like to:
- Have more energy?
- Be thinner?
- Sleep better?
- Lower your cholesterol and/or blood pressure?
- Get rid of your cravings for sweets?
- Think more clearly and remember more?
- Be less moody?
- Reduce your risk of heart disease and diabetes?
- Stay healthy and active as you age?
- Have more sex drive?
- Be stronger?
- Decrease joint pain?

Many individuals have achieved all of the above and more through simple lifestyle changes.

Lifestyle changes are vital and "first line" in protecting your health against an array of diseases including those of the heart, diabetes, arthritis, obesity and much more. In short, when your underlying cellular health is better, your energy levels are higher, your body metabolizes fat better, you lose unhealthy fat easier, your mental function is better, your sex drive is stronger, you sleep better… you just feel better all over!

According to the *Journal of the American Medical Association* "most physicians lack the time, information technology, and financial incentives to develop organized processes to systematically improve the quality of care provided to these patients (patients with chronic disease)."[2]

Furthermore, A scientific statement published in *Circulation* in 2004 called *Preventing Cancer, Cardiovascular Disease, and Diabetes; a Common Agenda for the American Cancer Society, the American Diabetes Association, and the American Heart Association,* states the following:[3]

- Cardiovascular disease (CVD), cancer, and diabetes account for nearly 2 of every 3 deaths.
- The cost is $700 billion per year.
- "While healthcare costs skyrocket, the national investment in prevention was estimated at less than 3 percent of the total annual healthcare expenditure."
- "Current approaches to health promotion and prevention of CVD, cancer and diabetes do not approach the potential of the existing state of knowledge."
- "Health care providers and medical organizations must transform this model into systems that provide preventive care and early detection as an integral part of standard medical practice."

It is also our individual responsibility to take charge of our health, become educated, and make choices that support a healthy lifestyle. If we choose not to take action, the life expectancy for obese men and women is shortened by 8 to 20 years.

Remember we are only as young as our oldest part.

The value of lifestyle changes in actual practice is often discounted by clinicians and health insurers who instead frequently turn to widely available pharmacotherapeutic agents: "Many patients with classic CVD risk factors can achieve risk reduction goals without medications within only three months of initiating therapeutic lifestyle changes."[4]

It is important to remember that lifestyle changes are also a family matter and that includes our children. Frighteningly, today 1 out of 6 adults have an obese child at home. What's worse, if a child is obese as a kindergartener and continues as an adult, he or she will have a decreased lifespan. According to the *New England Journal of Medicine* in 2005, compared to individuals who did not develop heart disease, those who were hospitalized for or died from coronary heart disease had relatively small body size during the first two years of life, and thereafter put on weight rapidly.

Of the obese children, 49 percent have metabolic syndrome (obesity, high triglycerides, high blood pressure, elevated blood glucose, and low HDL cholesterol) and are predicted to be disabled and die of cardiovascular disease in their 40's! This suggests that future generations may have shorter, less healthy lives if these current trends continue.[5]

Prevalence of obese children in the US:

Age Range	1980	2002
6–11 years	7%	16% (More than doubled)
12–19 years	5%	16% (More than tripled)

US Dept of Health and Human Services[6]

Healthy choices are a path to better health, increased energy and more success! Do not wait. The time to put your health first may never be "just right". Start where you are mentally and emotionally right now, and work with whatever tools you may have at your finger tips. Better and more effective tools will be developed as you progress.

You will not have a chance to experience healthy aging if you fall into one of the common and often fatal pitfalls that claim people in midlife. To avoid many common illnesses, you must be aware of your personal health risks as suggested by your past medical history, your family history, and medical examinations.

Today, specialized state-of-the art testing using organic acids and genetic testing is available to help complete your medical profile. Comprehensive health assessment and analysis can determine many types of energy imbalances within the human body such as food allergies, hormonal imbalances, environmental toxins, nutritional deficiencies, metabolic disturbances, underlying stress, and other imbalances that may be impacting our health.

Healthy Lifestyle Tips:

- Avoid what you already know is harmful.
- Maintain a normal healthy weight.
- Make good food choices:
  1. Avoid partially hydrogenated oil, trans fat, and margarine.
  2. Use cold pressed organic oils that are in dark glass containers otherwise they are oxidized and harmful.
  3. Avoid fried foods in restaurants as the oils may contain oxidized, damaged fats.
  4. Use extra-virgin olive oil.
  5. Eat less meat and poultry, more cold water fish.
  6. Eat more vegetable protein: legumes, nuts, and seeds.
  7. Choose organically grown foods.
  8. Increase fresh fruit and vegetables (6 to 8 servings a day).
- Eat 6 times a day: 3 small meals and 3 protein snacks.
- Walk, it is the best exercise:
  1. You already know how to do it.
  2. You can do it anywhere.
  3. It requires no equipment, just a good pair of shoes.
- Develop good sleeping habits:
  1. Get adequate rest.
  2. Sleep 8 hours.
- Touch and be touched—it is a basic requirement for optimum health. According to Jack Canfield daily hugs are vital to your health!
- Connect with nature, it is healing.
- Make your health a top priority.

- Take personal time for yourself.
- Decrease stress—it is essential not only to the quality of your life, but life itself.
- Laugh, love and have fun!

Dr. Andrew Weil, the father of integrative medicine, says, "Health is wholeness—wholeness in its most profound sense, with nothing left out and everything in just the right order to manifest the mystery of balance."

How do you find the right doctor? Unfortunately this can be difficult. Your friend says "he is a very nice doctor". First of all, being nice is a good thing. This does not mean he or she is any good.

The doctor has gone to the best schools, done research and is well published. So? Having practiced and taught in a major medical school and gone to school "forever", these criteria may mean nothing. I personally have been dismissed and misdiagnosed by many professionals in the medical and dental profession who look great on paper.

There are no easy answers, but here are a few thoughts. It makes sense that it would not be easy to find the right doctor for you. You are unique. You are putting your life in your doctor's hands. It has been said that we spend more time looking for a car or a dog than we do a doctor.

There are very few good quality measures available to assess individual doctors, so consumers must be prepared to do some research if they want to find a physician that can work with comfortably.

- What kind of care are you looking for? Primary care? OB/GYN?
- Google your list of potential doctors… but don't believe everything you read online.
- Make an appointment to meet the doctor for an interview. Ask the questions you want answers to. Ask if the doctor partners with his patients.
- Ask people you respect to recommend a physician. If they do not have a medical background it may not be the best source.
- Ask your doctor. Remember, the doctor may be referring to his friends, golf partners or members of his country club.

- Ask your doctor who his or her doctor is! Who does your doctor go to and who does he/she take his family to.

Here's a secret. Ask a *nurse* that works in the hospital. Nurses will often give you great recommendations as they "know" the doctors, have witnessed their skills, and their bedside manner.

Once you have chosen your doctor always keep copies of your complete medical record. Don't hesitate to look elsewhere, get second opinions, or change doctors if you are uncomfortable about their care or their communication with you. It's your right.

You deserve a physician who is highly qualified, someone with extensive experience who practices medicine with compassion. Education, caring, a life learner, and a good listener are important prerequisites.

> *"Change is the law of life. And those who look only to the past or present are certain to miss the future."*
> —John F. Kennedy, thirty-fifth President of the United States.

Todd is a 46 year old male who had suffered for years. Here is his story.

> *"I have had an extensive medical history that included multiple back, hip, and ankle surgeries. I was having concerns regarding my situation, my health, and my mental state during all of this. I was sitting at the doctor's office waiting to get another MRI when I picked up a natural health magazine. There was an advertisement from Dr. Norling's Mind Body Spirit Center. The ad asked, "are you tired of living in pain, not sleeping, etc…". I was at the end of my rope both physically and mentally. My wife urged me to make an appointment to see Dr. Norling."*
>
> *"Dr. Norling took an extensive survey, a number of lab tests, and put together a multifaceted plan to get me well. She changed my diet and provided me with natural supplements to get me back in order. In a matter of about a month, I was off all but two medications. I got off two hypertension meds, pain meds, anti-inflammatory meds, muscle relaxants, and sleep aids. I haven't felt this good in years."*

"I have had reduced pain levels, more energy, and a better state of mind. This better mental state was the most significant change that I and my family noticed. It affected everything regarding my attitude and how I am able to deal with my health situation. I developed a calmer positive outlook, reduced frustration levels, and increased tolerance in trying situations both at home and at work."

"I am also sleeping through most nights, which I haven't done in years. If you don't believe me ask my wife and children. They know how significant the changes have been. I am back to my old self. My wife has her husband back and my children have their dad back. As a matter of fact, whenever I experience a period of crankiness, they tell me to go back and see Dr. Norling."

"I want to conclude by saying that I no longer just exist. Life is no longer just an endless painful grind. I am living again and enjoying life as it should be lived. Thank you Dr. Norling for changing my life and bringing me back to the person, the father, and the husband I am meant to be." Todd.

- Your life can change forever. You and your family deserve you to have your best life.
- Health is our wealth and allows us to fully participate, enjoy and experience the best quality of life.
- Health is a resource that allows us to live the life we desire.
- Our daily choices affect how we experience life today and in the future.

Health makes your life worth living and your dreams come true.

You are not crazy. You are not making it up or suffering from a pharmaceutical drug deficiency. You can find the right doctor and find the root cause. You can feel better. You can be healthier and sexier.

It's not what has happened to you... It's what you do about it. There are only three choices in life. Give up. Give in. Give it all you've got.

The time is now.

Live your best life. You deserve it.

ABOUT THE AUTHOR

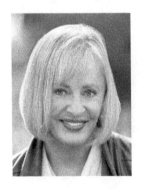

Sharon Norling, MD, MBA is a leading expert in functional medicine. As a medical doctor she is nationally board-certified in OB/GYN, Integrative Medicine and Medical Acupuncture. Dr Norling's life work has been to keep people healthy and safe.

Dr. Norling's expertise is based on her years of clinical experiences, her faculty position at the University of Minnesota Medical School, and her research. Importantly, she is a skilled and highly trained compassionate physician who finds the root cause of symptoms and illnesses. During her years in healthcare she has been nurse, medical doctor, hospital administrator, advocate and a dismissed and misdiagnosed patient.

She has testified before the White House Commission on Complementary Alternative Medicine Policy. She has served in multiple leadership roles as Medical Director and senior management in two large healthcare organizations. Her roles have brought her in direct contact with all levels of business, government and healthcare.

She is the author of numerous articles and co-author of the textbook, *Integrative Medicine.*

She founded the highly acclaimed Mind Body Spirit Center located in Westlake Village, CA, where she practices advanced medicine.

Dr. Sharon Norling is an international speaker on a wide range of current health topics, including corporate health. As a presenter, she is engaging, articulate, humorous, and insightful, making learning a dynamic professional and personal growth experience.

Whether you have heard on the radio, seen her on TV or sharing the stage with celebrities, Dr. Norling is the expert.

REFERENCES

Chapter 1

1. Hunt, Linda, PhD, et al. The Changing Face of Chronic Illness Management in Primary Care: A Qualitative Study of underlying Influences and Unintended Outcomes. *Annals of Family Medicine* September/October 2012

2. *Institute of Medicine*, www.iom.edu.; The Academy of Managed Care: Pharmacy's Control in Managed Care—website section on medication errors, www.amcp.org

3. Agency for Health Research and Quality 2001, www.ahrq.gov

4. Food and Drug Administration (FDA), www.fda.org

5. Kaushal R, Bates DW, Landrigan C, et al. Medication errors and adverse drug events in pediatric inpatients. *JAMA* 2001; 285:2114–2120. Thomas EJ, Brennan TA. Incidence and types of preventable adverse events in elderly patients: population based review of medical records. *BMF* 2000; 320:741–744.

6. Phillips J et al. Retrospective analysis of mortalities associated with medication errors. *American Journal of Health System-Pharmacy* Oct 2001; 58(19): 1835–41

7. Barker K.N. et al. Medication errors observed in 36 health care facilities. *Archives of Internal Medicine* 2002; 162:1897–1903.

8. Classen DC et al. Adverse drug events in hospitalized patients. *JAMA* 1997; 277:301–306. Lazarou J, Pomeranz BH, Corey PN. Incidence of adverse drug reaction in hospitalized patients. *JAMA* 1998; 279:1200–1205.

9. Lazarou J, Pomeranz BH, Corey PN. Incidence of adverse drug reactions in hospitalized patients: a meta-analysis of prospective studies. *JAMA*. 1998 Apr 15; 279(15): 1200–5.

10. Rabin R. Caution about overuse of antibiotics. *Newsday*. September 18, 2003.

11. Centers for Disease Control and Prevention. CDC antimicrobial resistance and antibiotic resistance—general information. Available at: http://www.cdc.gov/drugresistance/community/. Accessed December 13, 2003.

12. For calculations detail, see "Unnecessary Surgery." Sources: HCUPnet, Healthcare Cost and Utilization Project. Agency for Healthcare Research and Quality, Rockville, MD. Available at: http://www.ahrq.gov/data/hcup/hcupnet.htm. Accessed December 18, 2003. US Congressional House Subcommittee Oversight Investigation. *Cost and Quality of Health Care:Unnecessary Surgery* . Washington, DC: Government Printing Office; 1976. Cited in: McClelland GB, Foundation for Chiropractic Education and Research. Testimony to the Department of Veterans Affairs' Chiropractic Advisory Committee. March 25, 2003.

13. For calculations detail, see "Unnecessary Hospitalization." Sources: HCUPnet, Healthcare Cost and Utilization Project. Agency for Healthcare Research and Quality, Rockville, MD. Available at: http://www.ahrq.gov/data/hcup/hcupnet.htm. Accessed December 18, 2003. Siu AL, Sonnenberg FA, Manning WG, et al. Inappropriate use of hospitals in a randomized trial of health insurance plans. *N Engl J Med*. 1986 Nov 13; 315(20): 1259–66. Siu AL, Manning WG, Benjamin B. Patient, provider and hospital characteristics associated with inappropriate hospitalization. *Am J Public Health*. 1990 Oct; 80(10): 1253–6. Eriksen BO, Kristiansen IS, Nord E, et al. The cost

of inappropriate admissions: a study of health benefits and resource utilization in a department of internal medicine. *J Intern Med.* 1999 Oct; 246(4): 379–87.

14. Casalino, LP *Journal of the American Medical Association (JAMA)* 2005; 293: 485–488

15. Wu Sy, Green A. *Projection of Chronic Illness Prevalence and Cost Inflation.* Santa Monica, CA: Rand Health; 2000

16. Editors. *World Health Organization Publication.* September 2011

17. Sir William Osler, physician. *Aphorisms from his Bedside Teachings* 1961

18. Steering Committee of the Physicians' Health Study Research Group. *New England Journal of Medicine* July 20,1989; 321: 129–135

19. Food Additives and Contaminants May 2002. *Journal of Agricultural and Food Chemistry*, 2002, vol. 50(19); 2003, vol. 51(5)

20. Gillman MW, et al. Protective Effect of fruits and vegetables on development of stroke in men. JAMA 1995; 273: 1113–7. [PMID 7707599]

Chapter 2

1. Atkinson W, et al. Food elimination based on IgG antibodies in irritable bowel syndrome and randomized controlled trial. Department of Medicine, University Hospital of South Manchester, Manchester, UK; [PMID 15361495] PubMed—indexed for MEDLINE; *Gut* 2005; 54:566; BMJ Publishing Group LTD & British Society of Gastroenterology© 2005

2. Alessio Fasano, MD, et al. Prevalence of Celiac Disease in At-Risk and Not-At-Risk Groups in the U.S.: A Large Multicenter Study. *Archives of Internal Medicine* 2003; 163: 286–292

3. Biesiekierski J, et al. Gluten causes gastrointestinal symptoms in subjects without celiac disease: a double-blind randomized, placebo-controlled trial. *American Journal of Gastroenterology* March 2011; 106(3): 508–14

4. Ford A, et al. Yield of Diagnostic Tests for Celiac Disease in Individuals with Symptoms Suggestive of Irritable Bowel Syndrome: Review and Meta-Analysis. *Archives of Internal Medicine* April 13, 2009; Vol. 169, No. 7

5. Atkinson W, et al. Food elimination based on IgG antibodies in irritable bowel syndrome and randomized controlled trial. Department of Medicine, University Hospital of South Manchester, Manchester, UK; *Gut* October 2004; 53(10): 1459—64

Chapter 3

1. Current Trends in the Management of Gastroesophageal Reflux Disease: A Review. ISRN *Gastroenterol* 2012: 391631. Published online July 11, 2012 doi: 10.5402/2012/391631 [PMCID: PMC 3401535]
2. Gideon Lack, MD. Food Allergy. *New England Journal of Medicine* September 18, 2008; 359:1252–1260
3. Untersmayr E, et al. Antacid medication inhibits digestion of dietary proteins and causes food allergy. *Journal of Allergy and Clinical Immunology* 2003; 112: 616–623
4. Textbook for Functional Medicine; Institute for Functional Medicine; chapter 17, page 191
5. JAMA 2004; 292: 1955—1960. [PubMed 12]
6. Alan R. Gaby, MD and Jonathan V. Wright, MD. *Nutritional Therapy in Medical Practice: Reference Manual and Study Guide 2011 Edition*
7. Segal HL, Samloff IM. Gastric cancer—increased frequency in patients with achlorhydria.. PMID: 4695615 *American Journal of Digestive Diseases* April 1973; 18(4): 295–299.
8. Paul Schick, MD; Emmanuel C Besa. *Pernicious Anemia* Clinical Presentation. December 11, 2011
9. *The American Journal of Gastroenterology* January 2000; 157–165
10. https://www.consumerlab.com/reviews/Probiotic_Supplements_Including_Lactobacillus_acidophilus_Bifidobacterium_and_Others/probiotics/
11. M. Morisset, et al.; A Non-Hydrolyzed, Fermented Milk Formula Reduces Digestive and Respiratory Events in Infants at High Risk of Allergy. *European Journal of Clinical Nutrition* November 2010

Chapter 4

1. Women's Health Initiative Clinical Trial and Observational Study dbGaP Study Accession: phs000200.v7.p2 http://www.ncbi.nlm.nih.gov/projects/gap/

2. Rossouw, Jacques E et. al. Postmenopausal hormone therapy and risk of cardiovascular disease by age and years since menopause. *JAMA*: 2007; 297: 1465–77

3. *New England Journal of Medicine* 2007; Vol. 356: pp 2591–2602.

4. *British Medical Journal* August 2007; 335:239

5. *Journal of Clinical Endocrinology & Metabolism* 2011; 96: E1761–E1770;

6. *JAMA* 2011; 305: 1305–1314; 1354–1355

7. *The Lancet Oncology* May 2012; Vol. 13, Issue 5, Pp. 476—486

8. Francine Grodstein, Joann E. Manson, and Meir J. Stampfer. *Journal of Women's Health* January/February 2006; 15(1): 35–44

9. http://www.mayoclinic.org/news2009-mchi/5206.html

10. *Journal of Alzheimer's Disease* Vol. 6, No. 3/2004 Pp. 221–228

11. http://www.mayoclinic.com/health/bioidentical-hormones/AN01133

12. *International Journal of Cancer* October 2004; 20: 112(1): 130–4

13. Dessole S, Rubattu G, Ambrosini G et al. Efficacy of low-dose intravaginal estriol on urogenital aging in postmenopausal women. *Menopause* January 2004; 11(1): 49–56.

14. *Menopause: The Journal of The North American Menopause Society* 2007; Vol. 14, No. 2, pp. 168/182

15. *European Heart Journal* June 2010; 31(12): 1494–501 Epub 2010 Feb 17.

16. http://www.fda.gov/Drugs/DrugSafety/PostmarketDrugSafetyInformationforPatientsandProviders/ucm162862.htm

17. http://journals.lww.com/jneuro-ophthalmology/pages/collectiondetails.aspx?TopicalCollectionId=2

18. Carl J Lavie, MD, FACC. Vascular disease, hypertension, and prevention. *Journal of the American Colleges of Cardiology* 2004; 44(2s1): S19–S22. doi: 10.1016/j.jacc.2004.06.018

19. http://www.nih.gov/news/pr/aug2006/nhlbi-24.htm

20. http://www.cdc.gov/nutrition/downloads/r2p_life_change.pdf

21. A New Paradigm in Cardiovascular Disease Risk Reduction: Childhood Metabolic Syndrome *Marc Jacobson, MD* Disclosure: Dr. Ornstein has a modest Honoraria relationship with Pri-Med Institute; Dr. Jacobson has no conflicts. Pub Date: Monday, January 12, 2009 Author: Rollyn M Ornstein, MD

22. Buse JB, Ginsberg HN, Bakris GL, Clark NG, Costa F, Eckel R, et al. Primary prevention of cardiovascular diseases in people with diabetes mellitus: A scientific statement from the American Heart Association and the American Diabetes Association. *Circulation.* 2007; 115(1):114–126.

23. http://www.menopause.org/for-women/-i-menopause-flashes-i-/heart-health

24. http://www.nia.nih.gov/health/publication/whats-your-plate-smart-food-choices-healthy-aging/healthy-lifestyle-next-step

25. Morgentaler A. Testosterone for Life. New York: McGraw-Hill; 2008.

26. http://www.stocksinstitute.com/testosterone-and-prostate-cancer

Chapter 5

1. Lou Paget. *The Great Lover Playbook: 365 Sexual Tips and Techniques to Keep the Fires Burning All Year Long* January 13, 2005

2. Robert Fried and Lynn Edlen-Nezin *Great Food, Great Sex: The Three Food Factors for Sexual Fitness.* May 30, 2006

3. Andrea Salonia MD et al. *Original Research on Women's Sexual Health: Chocolate and Women's Sexual Health—An Intriguing Correlation.* Article first published online: February 27, 2006 doi: 10.1111/j.1743-6109.2006.00236.x

4. Yoshihiro Kamada et al. Vascular endothelial dysfunction resulting from L-arginine deficiency in a patient with lysinuric protein intolerance. Department of Internal Medicine and Molecular Science and School of Medicine, Osaka University, Osaka, Japan July 20, 2001

5. Hong B, J Urol et al.. A double-blind crossover study evaluating the efficacy of Korean red ginseng in patients with erectile dysfunction: a preliminary report. November 2002; 168(5): 2070–3; Department of

Urology, University of Ulsan College of Medicine, Asan Medical Center, Seoul, Korea.

6. Hirsch, A.R.. *Sexually Exciting Odors.* August/September, 2004; pp.14–15. Chicago Image

7. IU Health and Wellness: Study confirms exercise-induced orgasm; plus travel tips for teens. http://newsinfo.iu.edu/news/page/normal/21547.html

8. Marrena Lindberg. *The Orgasmic Diet: A Revolutionary Plan to Lift Your Libido and Bring You to Orgasm* by Crown Publishing division of Random House 2007

9. http://newsinfo.iu.edu/news/page/normal/21547.html

10. J. Dennis Fortenberry, M.D., professor at the IU School of Medicine and Center for Sexual Health Promotion. *Sexual and Relationship Therapy,* a leading peer-reviewed journal in the area of sex therapy and sexual health. http://newsinfo.iu.edu/news/page/normal/21547.html

11. Fay A. Guarraci, Anastasia Benson. *Coffee, Tea and Me:* Moderate doses of caffeine affect sexual behavior in female rats, Department of Psychology at Southwestern University, Georgetown, TX http://dx.doi.org/10.1016/j.pbb.2005.10.007

12. http://health.howstuffworks.com/sexual-health/sexual-dysfunction/top-10-natural-ways-to-boost-libido4.htm

13. Carl J. Charnetski and Francis X. Brennan. *Feeling Good Is Good for You: How Pleasure Can Boost Your Immune System and Lengthen Your Life* November 2003

14. Davey Smith G, Frankel S, Yarnell J. Sex and death: are they related? *British Medical Journal.* December 20, 1997; 315 (7123): 1641–4.

15. Burleson MH, Trevathan WR, Todd M. In the mood for love or vice versa? Exploring the relations among sexual activity, physical affection, affect, and stress in the daily lives of mid-aged women. *Archives of Sexual Behavior,* June 2007.

Chapter 6

1. Kessler RC et al. Prevalence, severity, and comorbidity of twelve-month DSM-IV disorders in the National Comorbidity Survey Replication (NCS-R). *Archives of General Psychiatry* June 2005; 62(6): 617–27

2. Kirsch I, Deacon BJ, et al. Initial Severity and Antidepressant Benefits: A Meta-Analysis of Data Submitted to the Food and Drug Administration. PLoS Medicine 2008; 5(2): e45.

3. Trivedi MH, Rush AJ, et al. Evaluation of Outcomes With Citalopram for Depression Using Measurement-Based Care in STAR*D: Implications for Clinical Practice. *American Journal of Psychiatry* 2006; 163: 28–40

4. Laura A. Pratt Ph.D et al. NCHS Data Brief Number 76, October 2011—Antidepressant Use in Persons Aged 12 and Over: United States, 2005–2008

5. Lazar SW et al. Meditation experience is associated with increased cortical thickness. *NeuroReport* 2005; 16:1893–1897.

6. Smith, Katharine A., MRCPsych et al. Impaired Regulation of Brain Serotonin Function during Dieting in Women Recovered from Depression. *The British Journal of Psychiatry* 2000: 72–75

7. Balcioglu A, Wurtman RJ. Effects of phentermine on striatal dopamine and serotonin release in conscious rats: in vivo microdialysis study. *International Journal of Obesity & Related Metabolic Disorders* 1998; 22: 325–328.

8. Arcaro, K. and D. C. Spink. Understanding the Human Health Effects of Chemical Mixtures. *Environmental Health Perspectives Supplement 2002* 110: S1

9. Wichers MC, Maes M. The role of indoleamine 2,3-dioxygenase (IDO) in the pathophysiology of interferon-alpha-induced depression. *Journal of Psychiatry and Neuroscience* January 2004; 29(1): 11–7

10. Brown D, Gaby AR, Reichert R. Natural Remedies for Depression. *Nutritional Science News* February 1999

11. R P Tracy. Emerging relationships of inflammation, cardiovascular disease and chronic diseases of aging. *International Journal of Obesity* 2003; 27: S29–S34

12. http://www.cdc.gov/nutrition/everyone/basics/protein.html

13. Young SN, Ghadirian AM.. Folic Acid and Psychopathology. *Progress in Neuro-Psychopharmacology and Biological Psychiatry* 1989; 13(6): 841–63.

14. Dietary Magnesium and C-reactive Protein Levels. *Journal of the American College of Nutrition* 2005; Vol. 24, No. 3, 166–171

15. Jaffe R MD. How to Know if You are Magnesium Deficient: 75% of Americans Are (transcript), June 16, 2005 www.innovativehealing.com

16. Holick, Michael F. Vitamin D Deficiency. *New England Journal of Medicine* 2007; 357: 266–281

17. Russell L. Blaylock, M.D. Key Points: *Blaylock Wellness Report* 2008 Vol. 5, No. 3

18. Gershon, Michael. *The Second Brain.* New York: HarperCollins, 1998.

19. Habib KE, Gold PW, Chrousos GP. Neuroendocrinology of stress. *Endocrinology Metabolism Clinics of North America* September 2001; 30(3): 695–728; vii–viii.

Chapter 7

1. David Perlmutter and Carol Colman. *The Better Brain Book* August 2005

2. Mary Shomon. *The High Cholesterol Thyroid Connection: Undiagnosed Thyroid Disease May Be the Reason for Your High Cholesterol* November 2009 http://www.nlm.nih.gov/medlineplus/ency/article/000403.htm

3. *Harvard Health Publications* in consultation with Jeffery R. Garber, M.D., Associate Professor of Medicine, Harvard Medical School 2012 http://www.health.harvard.edu/special_health_reports/thyroid-disease-understanding-hypothyroidism-and-hyperthyroidism

4. En-Ting Chang et al. Influence of L-Thyroxine Administration in Patients with Euthyroid Hashimoto's Thyroiditis. *Endocrine Society's Endo 2005 Abstracts*

5. Chu M, Seltzer TF. Myxedema coma induced by ingestion of raw bok choy. *New England Journal of Medicine* 2010; 362(20): 1945–1946.

6. James Wilson. *Adrenal Fatigue: The 21st Century Stress Syndrome* Smart Publications 2001; Petaluma, CA

7. Stress in America 2009. *American Psychological Association.* Retrieved from http://www.apa.org/news/press/releases/stress-exec-summary.pdf

8. The General Adaptation Syndrome and the Diseases of Adaptation. *The Journal of Clinical Endocrinology & Metabolism* February 1, 1946 vol. 6 no. 2 117–230; doi: 10.1210/jcem-6-2-117

Chapter 8

1. http://m.drugabuse.gov/publications/science-addiction/drug-abuse-addiction
2. http://www.drugabuse.gov/publications/drugfacts/treatment-statistics#sources
3. http://www.casacolumbia.org/upload/2012/20120626addictionmed.pdf
4. http://www.casacolumbia.org/articlefiles/379-Teen%20Tipplers.pdf
5. http://www.drugabuse.gov/publications/topics-in-brief/prescription-drug-abuse
6. The Journal of Neuroscience, October 15, 1999; 19(20): 9141–9148
7. Peter R. Breggin. Psychiatric drug-induced Chronic Brain Impairment (CBI): Implications for long-term treatment with psychiatric medication. *International Journal of Risk & Safety in Medicine. 2011; 23:* 193–200
8. http://psychcentral.com/lib/2006/what-is-sexual-addiction/
9. Under the Counter: The Diversion and Abuse of Controlled Prescription Drugs in the U.S. The National Center on Addiction and Substance Abuse at Columbia University, July 2005
10. http://www.casacolumbia.org/upload/2012/20120626addictionmed.pdf

Chapter 9

1. Thomas R. Dawber, M.D., Gilcin F. Meadors, M.D., M.P.H., and Felix E. Moore, Jr., *National Heart Institute, National Institutes of Health, Public Health Service, Federal Security Agency, Washington, D. C., Epidemiological Approaches to Heart Disease: The Framingham Study* Presented at a Joint Session of the Epidemiology, Health Officers, Medical Care, and Statistics Sections of the American Public Health Association. November 3, 1950.
2. J Rheumatol 2004; 31 Supplement 69:3–8
3. De Kort S., et.al. *Obesity Reviews* 2011; 12 (6): 449–58
4. Tsai F, et.al. *Gastroenterol Report* August 2009; 11(4): 307–13

5. Schober SE, et al. *Environmental Health Perspective* 114:1538–1541 (2006)

6. Menke A. et al. *Epub Circulation.* September 2006; 114(13): 1388–94. Blood lead below 0.48 micromol/L (10 microg/dL) and mortality among US adults. Department of Epidemiology, Tulane University, New Orleans, LA

7. Houston, MC, *Journal of Clinical Hypertension* August 2011; 13(8): 621–7

8. Houston, MC, *Therapeutic Advances in Cardiovascular Disease* June 2010; 4(3); 165–83.

9. Houston, MC, *Expert Review of Cardiovascular Therapy* June 2010; 8(6): 821–33

10. Lang I A, et.al. *JAMA* 2008; 300 (11) 1303–10

11. Jones O A, et.al. *Lancet* 2008; 371 (9609): 287–8

12. Alessandra D., Fisher MD. Sexual and Cardiovascular Correlates of Male Unfaithfulness, Article first published online: April 17, 20–12. *The Journal of Sexual Medicine* June 2012; Vol. 9, Issue 6, pp. 1508–1518

13. Glenn N. Levine, MD, FAHA, Elaine E. Steinke, RN, PhD, FAHA. Scientific Statement Sexual Activity and Cardiovascular Disease A Scientific Statement From the American Heart Association; American Heart Association Council on Clinical Cardiology, Council on Cardiovascular Nursing, Council on Cardiovascular Surgery and Anesthesia, and Council on Quality of Care and Outcomes Research *Circulation. 2012; 125: 1058–1072* Published online before print January 19, 2012, doi: 10.1161/CIR.0b013e3182447787

14. Alessandra D. Fisher MD et al. Sexual and Cardiovascular Correlates of Male Unfaithfulness. *The Journal of Sexual Medicine* June 2012; Vol. 9, Issue 6, pp. 1508–1518

15. English KM et al. Low-dose transdermal testosterone improves angina threshold in men with chronic stable angina. *Circulation* 2000; 102 (16): 1906–11.

16. Kupelian V. et al. Low sex hormone binding globulin, total testosterone, and androgen deficiency are associated with development of the

metabolic syndrome in non-obese men. *Journal of Clinical Endocrinology and Metabolism* 2006; 91: 843–50.

17. Oh JY et al. Endogenous sex hormones and the development of type 2 diabetes in older men and women: The Rancho Bernardo study. *Diabetes Care* 2002; 25:55–60

18. Malkin CJ et al: The effect of testosterone replacement on endogenous inflammatory cytokines and lipid profiles in hypogondal men. *Journal of Clinical Endocrinology & Metabolism* July 2004; 89(7): 3313–8.

19. Malkin CJ et al. Testosterone replacement in hypogonadal men with angina improves ischemic threshold and quality of life. *Heart* August 2004; 90(8): 871–6.

20. Intermountain Medical Center Treating vitamin D deficiency significantly reduces heart disease risk. March 17, 2010

21. Leslie Cho, MD, Cleveland Clinic Cardiologist. *Circulation.* 2008; 117:503–511

22. IMS Health. US top ten products by prescriptions http://www.imshealth.com/public/structure/dispcontent/1,2779,1343-1343-144004,00.html [April 19, 2001]

23. National Prescription Audit Plus™. *IMS Health* 2002; Lipitor leads the way in 2003. URL: http://www.ims-global.com/insight/news_story/0403/news_story_040316.htm. [Accessed May 23, 2005]

24. *IMS Health.* IMS global insights. IMS Retail Drug Monitor 2007; URL: http://www.imshealth.com/web/content/0,3148,64576068_63872702_70260998_83746585,00.html [Accessed May 2, 2008]

25. http://www.ama-assn.org/amednews/2004/11/01/hlsa1101.htm

26. Cardiovascular Therapeutic Drugs: Technologies and Global Markets *BCC Research* July 1, 2010

27. Rundek T et al. Atorvastatin decreases the coenzyme Q10 level in the blood of patients at risk for cardiovascular disease and stroke. *Archives of Neurology* June 2004; 61(6): 889–92. Department of Neurology, Columbia University College of Physicians & Surgeons, New York, NY

28. Beatrice A. Golomb; Marcella A. Evans. Statin Adverse Effects: A Review of the Literature and Evidence for a Mitochondrial Mechanism. *American Journal of Cardiovascular Drugs* 2008; 8(6): 373–418.

29. U.S. Department of Health and Human Services, National Institutes of Health National Heart, Lung, and Blood Institute *NIH Publication* December 2005 No.06–5235

30. Jennifer L. Jones, PhD et al. A Mediterranean-style low-glycemic-load diet improves variables of metabolic syndrome in women, and addition of a phytochemical-rich medical food enhances benefits on lipoprotein metabolism. *Journal of Lipidology* January 2011; page 197

31. Paul M Ridker, MD. Number Needed to Treat With Rosuvastatin to Prevent First Cardiovascular Events and Death Among Men and Women With Low Low-Density Lipoprotein Cholesterol and Elevated High-Sensitivity C-Reactive Protein Justification for the Use of statins in Prevention: an Intervention Trial Evaluating Rosuvastatin (JUPITER Study Group) *Circoutcomes* 2009; 109.848473 Published online. doi: 10.1161/circoutcomes.109.848473

32. Machan, Carolyn M.; Hrynchak, Patricia K.; Irving, Elizabeth L. Age-Related Cataract Is Associated with Type 2 Diabetes and Statin Use. *Optometry & Vision Science* August 2012; 89(8): 1165–1171; doi: 10.1097/OPX.0b013e3182644cd1

33. Culver A L et. al. *Archives of Internal Medicine* 2012; 172 (2): 144–52

34. Jacobs DR, Blackburn H, Higgins M, Reed D, Iso H, McMillan G, et al. Report of the conference on low blood cholesterol: mortality associations. *Circulation* 1992; 86:1046–1060.

35. Persson IA et al. Effects of cocoa extract and dark chocolate on angiotensin-converting enzyme and nitric oxide in human endothelial cells and healthy volunteers—a nutrigenomics perspective. *Journal of Cardiovascular Pharmacology* January 2011; 57(1): 44–50. Division of Pharmacology, Department of Medical and Health Sciences, Faculty of Health Sciences, Linkoping University, Linköping, Sweden

36. Cardiovascular Perspectives JUPITER A Few Words of Caution Viola Vaccarino, MD, PhD, J. Douglas Bremner, MD and Mary E. Kelley,

PhD *Circulation: Cardiovascular Quality and Outcomes. 2009; 2: 286–288*

37. Genest J et al. Lipoprotein cholesterol, apolipoprotein A-1 and B and lipoprotein (a) abnormalities in men with premature coronary artery disease. *Journal of the American College of Cardiology* 1992; 19: 792–802.

38. Reaven GM, Chen YD, Jeppesen J, Maheux P, Krauss RM. Insulin resistance and hyperinsulinemia in individuals with small, dense low-density lipoprotein particles. *Journal of Clinical Investigation* July 1993; 92(1): 141–146.

39. Michael Cobble, MD. Atherotech Laboratories Clinically Meaningful Underestimation of LDL-C by Friedewald at Levels Below 70 mg/dL: A Study of 1.3 Million Adults—Very Large Database of Lipids (VLDL). Seth Martin, MD, et al. Poster presented at the American College of Cardiology—Scientific Sessions March 2012—Current Research in Lipidology.http://www.atherotech.com/images/vapliterature/pdfs/ACC%20MAB%20Poster%2021Mar12.pdf

40. Vascular disease, hypertension, and prevention FREE Carl J Lavie, MD, FACC *J Am Coll Cardiol.* 2004; 44(2s1): S19–S22. doi: 10.1016/j.jacc.2004.06.018

41. http://www.nih.gov/news/pr/aug2006/nhlbi-24.htm

42. http://www.cdc.gov/nutrition/downloads/r2p_life_change.pdf

43. A New Paradigm in Cardiovascular Disease Risk Reduction: Childhood Metabolic Syndrome *Marc Jacobson, MD* Disclosure: Dr. Ornstein has a modest Honoraria relationship with Pri-Med Institute; Dr. Jacobson has no conflicts. Pub Date: Monday, January 12, 2009 Author: Rollyn M Ornstein, MD

44. Buse JB, Ginsberg HN, Bakris GL, Clark NG, Costa F, Eckel R, et al. Primary prevention of cardiovascular diseases in people with diabetes mellitus: A scientific statement from the American Heart Association and the American Diabetes Association. *Circulation.* 2007; 115(1): 114–126.

45. http://www.menopause.org/for-women/-i-menopause-flashes-i-/heart-health

46. http://www.nia.nih.gov/health/publication/whats-your-plate-smart-food-choices-healthy-aging/healthy-lifestyle-next-step

Chapter 10

1. Broad scan analysis of the FY82 national human adipose tissue survey specimens. EPA Office of Toxic Substances. EPA 560/5-86-035

2. http://www.ewg.org/reports/bodyburden2/execsumm.php

3. http://www.fda.gov/ForConsumers/ConsumerUpdates/ucm294849.htm

4. http://www.ewg.org/skindeep/top-tips-for-safer-products/

5. http://www.ewg.org/skindeep/

6. Kays Kaidbey et al. AHAs enhance UV-induced damage to DNA in the skin Topical glycolic acid enhances photodamage by ultraviolet light, *Photodermatology, Photoimmunology and Photomedicine* 2003; vol.19, issue 1, pp. 21–27

7. http://www.ewg.org/skindeep/myths-on-cosmetics-safety/

8. Houlihan, J., Wiles, R., Thayer, K. & Gray S. *Body burden: The pollution in people June 15, 2003* http://archive.ewg.org/reports/bodyburden1/pdf/BBreport_final.pdf

9. Cosmetics with banned and unsafe ingredients. Table 1—Banned in other countries. Accessed June 21, 2010. EWG (Environmental Working Group) 2007b. http://www.ewg.org/node/22624

10. Cosmetics With Banned and Unsafe Ingredients. Table 2—Unsafe for use in cosmetics, according to industry. Accessed June 21, 2010. EWG (Environmental Working Group). 2007c. http://www.ewg.org/node/22636.

11. EWG Comments to FDA on Nano-Scale Ingredients in Cosmetics. Docket: FDA Regulated Products Containing Nanotechnology Materials. EWG (Environmental Working Group). 2006. Docket number: 2006N-0107. http://www.ewg.org/node/21738

12. EWG research shows 22 percent of cosmetics may be contaminated with cancer-causing impurity. EWG (Environmental Working Group). 2007d. http://www.ewg.org/node/21286

13. EWG's 2010 sunscreen guide. Nano-materials and hormone disruptors in sunscreens. EWG (Environmental Working Group) 2010. http://www.ewg.org/2010sunscreen/full-report/nanomaterials-and-hormone-disruptors-in-sunscreens/

14. Calafat AM, Wong LY, Ye X, Reidy JA, Needham LL. 2008. Concentrations of the sunscreen agent benzophenone-3 in residents of the United States: National Health and Nutrition Examination Survey 2003–2004. Environ Health Perspect. 2008 Jul; 116(7):893–7.

15. CSC (Campaign for Safe Cosmetics) 2007. Lead in lipstick. http://www. safecosmetics.org/article.php?id=223

16. Valarie Natale. BCC Report Code—PHM037B, Published May 2008

17. Certech Registration Inc. 2008. International organic standard—Natural and natural organic cosmetic certification. *IOS Cosmetics.* Issue 01, April 2008 http://www.certechregistration.com/IOS_cosmetics_standard.pdf

18. Carol Lewis. FDA (U.S. Food and Drug Administration). 1998. Clearing Up Cosmetic Confusion. *FDA Consumer Magazine.* May–June 1998. http://www.pueblo.gsa.gov/cic_text/health/cosmetic-confusion/398_cosm.html

19. Safety Guide to Children's Personal Care Products. EWG (Environmental Working Group). 2007a. http://www.ewg.org/skindeep/special/parentsguide/summary.php

20. FDA (U.S. Food and Drug Administration). 2005. FDA authority over cosmetics. http://www.cfsan.fda.gov/dms/cos-206.html

21. http://notjustaprettyface.org/

22. Autier P et al. Sunscreen use, wearing clothes, and number of nevi in 6- to 7-year-old European children. *Journal of the National Cancer Institute* 1998; 90: 1873–80

23. Beitner H et al. Malignant melanoma: aetiological importance of individual pigmentation and sun exposure. Br. 1. *Dermatology* 1990; 122: 43–51

24. Sunscreen use and malignant melanoma. *International Journal of Cancer* July 2000; 1; 87(1): 145–50. Westerdahl J, Ingvar C, Måsbäck A, Olsson H. Source Department of Surgery, University Hospital, Lund, Sweden

25. Fink-Puches R, Soyer HP, Hofer A, Kerl H, Wolf P. Long-term follow-up and histological changes of superficial non-melanoma skin cancers treated with topical delta-aminolevulinic acid photodynamic therapy. *Archives of Dermatology* 1998; 134(7): 821–826

26. Barr, L. et al. Measurement of paraben concentrations in human breast tissue at serial locations across the breast from axilla to sternum. *Journal of Applied Toxicology.* ISSN 1099-1263

27. Mannello F, et al. Analysis of aluminum content and iron homeostasis in nipple aspirate fluids from healthy women and breast cancer-affected patients. *Journal of Applied Toxicology* Feb 21, 2011

28. Hepp, N.M. Determination of Total Lead in 400 Lipsticks on the U.S. Market Using a Validated Microwave-Assisted Digestion, Inductively Coupled Plasma–Mass Spectrometric Method. *Journal of Cosmetic Science* May/June 2012

29. CDC. Infant Lead Poisoning Associated with Use of Tiro, an Eye Cosmetic from Nigeria. Boston, Massachusetts, 2011. *MMWR.* August 3, 2012 61(30); 574–576

30. Washington Post Published: January 30, 2012 http://www.washingtonpost.com/national/health-science/soaps-makeup-and-other-items-contain-deadly-ingredients-say-consumer-advocates/2012/01/24/gIQAeJ56cQ_story.html

31. http://www.ewg.org/skindeep/top-tips-for-safer-products/

32. http://www.johnsonsbaby.com/a-statement-on-ingredients-in-the-news/

33. *Monographs on the Evaluation of Carcinogenic Risks to Humans Volume 88 (2006): Formaldehyde, 2-Butoxyethanol and 1-tert-Butoxypropan-2-ol. International Agency for Research on Cancer* June 2004. http://monographs.iarc.fr/ENG/Monographs/vol88/index.php

34. http://www.ewg.org/skindeep/top-tips-for-safer-products/

35. http://www.ewg.org/skindeep/ingredient/706623/TRICLOSAN/

36. State of California Environmental Protection Agency Office of Environmental Health Hazard Assessment Safe Drinking Water and Toxic Enforcement Act of 1986 Chemicals Known to the State to Cause Cancer or Reproductive Toxicity—April 2, 2010

37. Plastics leach toxic substances; *The Hindu* 2011; University of Gothenburg

38. Frederick S. vom Saal, PhD; John Peterson Myers, PhD. Bisphenol A and Risk of Metabolic Disorders *JAMA.* September 17, 2008; 008: 300(11): 1353–1355.

39. *International Agency for Research on Cancer* (IARC) Monographs, 29 CFR 1910 subpart Z, OSHA Toxic & Hazardous Substances

40. *International Agency for Research on Cancer* (IARC)—Summaries & Evaluations STYRENE (Group 2B) 2002; Vol 82, p. 437, Case No. 100-42–5

41. http://www.aaidd.org/ehi/media/polluting_report.pdf

42. *FDA Consumer Magazine* May–June 2004 http://www.chifountain.com/ studies_Folder/MercuryJune04.pdf

43. Children's Health and the Environment Training Package for the Health Sector World Health Organization (WHO) www.who.int/ceh. Training for the Health Sector, July 2008

44. Pesticide Data Program Annual Summary, 2009; United States Department of Agriculture / Agricultural Marketing Service Science and Technology Programs www.ams.usda.gov/pdp

45. http://www.ewg.org/foodnews/list/

46. Chester, D.N., Goldman, J.D., Ahuja, J.K., Moshfegh, A.J. 2011. Dietary intakes of choline: What We Eat In America, *NHANES* 2007–2008. www.ars.usda.gov/Services/docs.html?docid=19476

47. http://action.ewg.org/p/dia/action/public/?action_KEY=1956&tag= 2012GMOLongVActionTaker&utm_source=gmo2012longv&utm_ medium=email&utm_content=second-link&utm_campaign=food

48. 2010 TRI National Analysis Overview http://www.epa.gov/tri/tridata/ tri10/nationalanalysis/overview/2010TRINAOverview.pdf

49. http://www.fsis.usda.gov/FACTSheets/Additives_in_Meat_&_Poultry_ Products/index.asp

50. http://www.usda.gov/wps/portal/usda/usdahome?navid=SEARCH&mod e=simple&q=pesticides+and+herbicides+we+eat&x=0&y=0&site=usda

51. The Essential Phospholipids as a Membrane Therapeutic

52. Publisher: *Polish Section of European Society of Biochemical Pharmacology* Institute of Pharmacology and Toxicology, Medical Academy, Szczecin 1993

53. Gold L. S. Slone, T.H. and Ames B.N. (1997a) Prioritization of possible carcinogenic hazards in food. *Food Chemical Risk Analysis* (D. R.

Tennant, ed.) pp. 267–295. Chapman & Hall, London http://potency.berkeley.edu/text/maff.html

54. http://www.aad.org/media-resources/stats-and-facts/conditions/hair-loss

55. Scientific Review and Clinical Applications | June 19, 2002 Clinician's Corner Vitamins for Chronic Disease Prevention in Adults Scientific Review Kathleen M. Fairfield, MD, DrPH; Robert H. Fletcher, MD, MSc *JAMA*. 2002; 287(23): 3116–3126.

Chapter 11

1. Blumenthal JA, et al. Department of Psychiatry and Behavioral Sciences, Duke University medical Center, Durham, NC. Effects of exercise training on older patients with depression. *Archives of Internal Medicine* October 25, 1999; 159(19); 2349–56.

2. Lawrence Casalino, MD, PhD; et al, *JAMA*. 2003; 289(4): 434–441

3. Eyre H, et al. Preventing cancer, cardiovascular disease and diabetes: a common agenda for the American Cancer Society, the American Diabetes Association and the American Heart Association. Circulation June 29, 2004; 109(25): 3244–55. Epub June 15, 2004

4. The American College of Cardiology Guidelines. http://www.cardiosource.org/science-and-quality

5. Centers for Disease Control and Prevention. http://www.cdc.gov/healthyyouth/obesity/facts.htm

6. U.S. Department of Health and Human Services 2011; http://www.cdc.gov/nchs/data/databriefs/db82.pdf

RESOURCES

Books

The Disease Delusion—Dr. Jeffrey S. Bland

The Blood Sugar Solution—Dr. Mark Hyman

What Your Doctor May Not Tell You about Heart Diseases—Dr. Mark Houston

The Success Principles—Jack Canfield

Grain Brain —Dr. David Perlmutter

Eight Weeks to Vibrant Health—Dr. Hyla Cass

Testosterone for Life: Recharge Your Vitality, Sex Drive, Muscle Mass, and Overall Health—Dr. Abraham Morgentaler

Laboratory Services

Cyrex Labs—www.cyrexlabs.com

Genova Diagnostics—www.gdx.net

Sanesco —www.sanescohealth.com/

Doctor's Data—www.doctorsdata.com/home.asp

Additional Resources

Dr. Sharon Norling—www.drsharonnorling.com

Dr. Sharon Norling—www.solutions4symptoms.com

Personalized Lifestyle Medicine Institute—www.plminstitute.org

Institute for Functional Medicine—www.functionalmedicine.org

Blue Zones—www.bluezones.com

Dr. David Perlmutter—www.drperlmutter.com

Dr. Mark Hyman—The UltraWellness Center—www.drhyman.com

Vitamin Angels—www.vitaminangels.org

Functional Medicine Clinical Research Center (FMCRC)—www.metagenics. com

American Board of Integrative Holistic Medicine—http://www.abihm.org

Forever Health—http://www.foreverhealth.com

DON'T WASTE ANOTHER DAY!

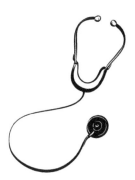

Go To:

http://drsharonnorling.com/your-doctor-is-wrong-bonus-page/

You Will Get:

- Free E-book: SEX: What Makes Woman Want More
- 5 keys to finding the root cause of your symptoms
- Webinar: How to be Happy, Energetic and Productive!
- + A very special surprise gift!

MAKE YOUR NEXT EVENT UNFORGETTABLE!

Dr. Norling is an internationally-renowned, dynamic speaker whose medical knowledge is well-respected and in high demand. As a presenter, she is engaging, articulate, humorous, insightful and memorable. As the author of *Your Doctor is Wrong* she draws large audience.

Dr. Norling's expertise is based on her years of clinical experiences, her faculty position at the University of Minnesota Medical School, and her research. Her roles have brought her in direct contact with all levels of business, government and healthcare. Recognized for her expertise, Dr. Norling has testified before the White House Commission on Complementary and Alternative Medicine Policy.

Importantly, she is a skilled and highly trained compassionate physician who finds the root cause of symptoms and illnesses. During her years in healthcare she has been nurse, medical doctor, hospital administrator, advocate and a dismissed and misdiagnosed patient.

Whether you have heard on the radio, seen her on TV or sharing the stage with celebrities, Dr. Norling is the expert. When she is speaking at conferences, groups, organizations, special events, or for corporations, she delivers a powerful keynote. Each presentation is customized. Her many health topics will resonate with everyone in the audience.

These are just some of the topics:

- Finding the Root Cause of Your Symptoms
- How to be Energetic, Focused and Happy
- Corporate Health—to Increase Your Bottom Line
- Hormones—Happiness, Health or Harm?
- Sex. What Makes Women Want More
- 3 Simple Steps to Get Rid of Pain and Brain Fog
- Addictions: What You Need to Know
- The New You—Restored and Regenerated
- Are You Sick and Tired of Being Sick and Tired?
- Are the Foods You are Eating Making You Sick?
- 5 Keys to Reversing Aging
- Low Testosterone—What You Need to Know May Save Your Life

Give your audience the gift of health and laughter!
Call now to have Dr. Norling present at your next event!
Phone: 818-707-9355
Fax 818-707-7255
www.drsharonnorlingpresents.com

Printed in the USA
CPSIA information can be obtained
at www.ICGtesting.com
JSHW022329140824
68134JS00019B/1380